Practical Laparoscopy

Practical Laparoscopy

ALAN G. GORDON FRCS, FRCOG
Honorary Consultant Gynaecologist,
Princess Royal Hospital, Hull, UK

AND

PATRICK J. TAYLOR MD, FRCS(C), FRCOG
Chairman of Department of Obstetrics & Gynaecology,
St Paul's Hospital, Vancouver,
and Professor of Obstetrics & Gynaecology,
University of British Columbia,
Vancouver, Canada

WITH A CHAPTER BY
CHRISTOPHER M.S. ROYSTON FRCS
& WILLIAM BROUGH FRCS

FOREWORD BY
CARL J. LEVINSON MD

WITH THE COMPLIMENTS OF
Karl Storz

OXFORD
Blackwell Scientific Publications
LONDON EDINBURGH BOSTON
MELBOURNE PARIS BERLIN VIENNA

© 1993 by
Blackwell Scientific Publications,
Editorial Offices:
Osney Mead, Oxford OX2 0EL
25 John Street, London, WC1N 2BL
23 Ainslie Place, Edinburgh EH3 6AJ
238 Main Street, Cambridge
  Massachusetts 02142, USA
54 University Street, Carlton
  Victoria 3053, Australia

Other Editorial Offices:
Librairie Arnette SA
2, rue Casimir-Delavigne
75006 Paris
France

Blackwell Wissenschafts-Verlag GmbH
Meinekestrasse 4
D-1000 Berlin 15
Germany

Blackwell MZV
Feldgasse 13
A-1238 Wien
Austria

First published 1993

Set by Semantic Graphics Services,
Singapore
Printed and bound in Great Britain
at the University Press,
Cambridge

DISTRIBUTORS

Marston Book Services Ltd
PO Box 87
Oxford OX2 0DT
(*Orders*: Tel: 0865 791155
    Fax: 0865 791927
    Telex: 837515)

USA
Blackwell Scientific Publications, Inc.
238 Main Street
Cambridge, MA 02142
(*Orders*: Tel: 800 759–6102
    617 876–7000)

Canada
Times Mirror Professional Publishing,
Ltd
130 Flaska Drive
Markham, Ontario L6G 1B8
(*Orders*: Tel: 800 268–4178
    416 470–6739)

Australia
Blackwell Scientific Publications Pty Ltd
54 University Street
Carlton, Victoria 3053
(*Orders*: Tel: 03 347–5552)

A catalogue record for this title
is available from the British Library

ISBN 0-632-03658-3

Library of Congress
Cataloging in Publication Data

Gordon, Alan G.
    Practical laparoscopy/Alan G.
Gordon and Patrick J. Taylor; with a
contribution by Christopher Royston;
foreword by Carl Levinson.
        p.   cm.
    Companion v. to: Practical
hysteroscopy/Patrick J. Taylor and
Alan G. Gordon
    Includes bibliographical references
    and index.
    ISBN 0-632-03709-1
    1. Laparoscopic surgery.
I. Taylor, Patrick J.   II. Royston,
Christopher.   III. Taylor, Patrick J.
Practical hysteroscopy.   IV. Title.
    [DNLM: 1. Peritoneoscopy.   WI
575 G662p 1993]
RG104.7.G67   1993
617'.05—dc20

Contents

Foreword

CARL J. LEVINSON*

What a pleasure it is to have a book such as this: not a lengthy article making a salient point inherent in the larger picture; not a tome of such ponderous nature that one can neither read it for enjoyment as well as for information, nor be able to find the information sought before forgetting what the purpose was; not a review of all the currently available techniques without opinion as to relative merit; and certainly not an imperative 'This is the only way it can be done correctly'. To put it in a more positive fashion, this is the book which will refresh your memory as to potential complications (in case your most recent operative procedure has not already done so); the book to refurbish your mind, quickly and easily regarding the principles that are important for either diagnostic or operative laparoscopy and to appreciate the difference.

This book represents the collaboration of two most experienced individuals covering somewhat less than two generations. The overlapping years bring with them the memories of the 'early years' of experimentation, trial and error and the complications of the 'learning curve'. Subsequent years bring a stage of standardization, firm development, a more routine educational process and, eventually, a large body of experience gathered from throughout the world—and that persistent wonderful view of 'pushing the boat out' still further.

How lucky the reader of this book: to have the learning process, the principles, the techniques, the complications, the results ... all distilled and as crystal clear as a distending medium should be. The reader is guaranteed that whether it is a panoramic view or a close-up of a specific area, this book will provide the subject with precision and clarity. Read on!

* Director, Stanford Endoscopy Center for Training & Technology and Associate Professor, Department of Gynaecology & Obstetrics, Stanford University School of Medicine, San Francisco, California, USA.

Preface

Until recently laparoscopy was used by most gynaecologists primarily for diagnostic procedures and for the performance of tubal sterilization. The last few years have seen enormous advances in our ability to use the laparoscope as a means of access to the abdominal and pelvic cavities to carry out advanced surgery both in gynaecology and other branches of surgery. The authors are grateful to their colleagues Christopher Royston and William Brough whose chapter on general surgery illustrates how laparoscopy has revolutionized the practice of their discipline. The saving to patients both in discomfort and the time necessary for hospitalization and return to normal activities are considerable. Fiscal advantages accrue to those who must pay for health care. Many of these procedures have been developed since practising gynaecologists and surgeons finished their training. They must now acquire these new skills and ensure that endoscopic surgery becomes an integral part of the experience of their junior staff.

This book and its companion *Practical Hysteroscopy*, have been written to serve as guides for clinicians who wish to develop their endoscopic skills. It is hoped that they will provide solid didactic foundations for those undertaking further training.

A.G.G., P.J.T.

Acknowledgements

The authors wish to express their appreciation for technical assistance to the following companies: Ethicon Ltd, Bank Head Avenue, Edinburgh EH11 4HE, UK, and Karl Storz GmbH, Mittelstrasse 8, 7200 Tuttlingen, Germany.

1: Introduction

Modern gynaecological endoscopy commenced in the early 19th century with Bozzini's attempts to examine the urethra of a living subject. For his pains he was censured by the Medical Faculty of the University of Vienna for showing 'undue curiosity'. Some 50 years later Panteleoni performed the first hysteroscopy on a woman with uterine polyps which he was able to cauterize. While hysteroscopy was practised half a century before laparoscopy, uterine distension was difficult to achieve without provoking bleeding which inevitably obscured vision. Hysteroscopy, therefore, did not become accepted and popular until many years later when these problems had been resolved.

Laparoscopy was not attempted until the early 20th century when the first operations were performed on dogs using air as the distension medium. Despite the crude nature of the instruments of that time, Jacobeus in Sweden reported performing 17 laparoscopies on human patients with ascites in 1912.

For the next 20 years laparoscopy was a procedure used almost solely by physicians to investigate abdominal tuberculosis and liver disease. The first recorded laparoscopic operation was by Fervers, a general surgeon, in 1933. He performed adhesiolysis using an electric current with oxygen as the distending medium. Oxygen, of course, supports combustion. He described vividly the flashes of light and the audible explosion within the abdomen and went on to say that 'it caused us great concern'. The general surgeons then appear to have abandoned the laparoscope for the next 50 years!

Gynaecological laparoscopy commenced in 1936, when Hope used the technique to diagnose an ectopic pregnancy. This was soon followed by the early sterilization operations using tubal fulgaration. Laparoscopy remained an essentially diagnostic tool until the last two decades when its potential as a means of access to perform surgical operations began to be realized. The development of bipolar electrocoagulation, endotherm and laser has increased the scope of surgery and improved its safety. In the last five years, new technology with clips, staples and suturing techniques has led to a huge development of interest in the possibilities of laparoscopic surgery. Infertility surgery, the treatment of endometriosis and pelvic inflammatory disease are now best performed by laparoscopy. Other more

1

advanced operations including myomectomy, hysterectomy and pelvic lymphadenectomy are becoming increasingly popular.

The wheel has turned a full circle for the general surgeon. After half a century of ignoring the possibilities of the laparoscope, the surgeons are performing cholecystectomy, appendicectomy, herniorrhaphy, vagotomy, bowel surgery and also many forms of urological surgery. The obituary to laparotomy has not only to be written, it is a reality. Some 70–80% of all intra-abdominal surgery may now be performed through incisions no longer than one centimetre.

This book is intended to provide the trainee with a step by step programme in learning the techniques of diagnostic and operative laparoscopy. Emphasis is placed throughout on the importance of training and the avoidance of complications. The reader should find in these pages a comprehensive guide to the safe and satisfying performance of laparoscopic surgery.

2: Instruments

Introduction

A range of instruments has been developed for diagnostic laparoscopy to allow safe inspection of the abdominal and pelvic viscera. They include the instruments used to produce a pneumoperitoneum, light sources, cables, and telescopes with high resolution lens systems to enable accurate examination with a clear, undistorted image. In addition, an ever increasing range of ancillary instruments enables therapeutic procedures to be performed using the laparoscope to gain access to the peritoneal cavity. Ability to manipulate the uterus and, where necessary, perform chromopertubation is usually a prerequisite of gynaecological laparoscopy. Effective performance of modern laparoscopic surgery demands the use of high resolution closed circuit television (CCTV).

Instruments for diagnostic laparoscopy

Diagnostic laparoscopy entails the production of a pneumoperitoneum to create space in which to work safely. The laparoscope is inserted through a cannula. Illumination is provided by an external light source and transmitted through fibreoptic cables to the telescope. Diagnostic laparoscopy cannot be performed effectively unless a probe is introduced with which to displace and manipulate the pelvic organs.

Distension media

The peritoneal cavity is normally only a potential space with the intra-abdominal and pelvic organs in contact with one another. It is essential, therefore, to distend the abdomen to make room into which instruments may be inserted to visualize the abdominal contents. In diagnostic laparoscopy a gaseous distension medium is used.

Carbon dioxide (CO_2) or nitrous oxide (N_2O) may be used. In the early days of laparoscopy, air or oxygen were common distension gases. Air is composed of nitrogen (79%) and oxygen (21%). Nitrogen is relatively insoluble in body fluids, is not resorbed for several days and therefore may lead to prolonged subphrenic discomfort. In addition, there is an unacceptable risk of causing fatal gas embolism. Oxygen was used in the 1930s but, while it is non-flammable, it supports combustion and therefore its use is dangerous in conjunction with electrosurgery.

Carbon dioxide

Carbon dioxide is an odourless, non-toxic gas which is 20 times more soluble in blood and body fluids than air or oxygen. It is inert and does not support combustion. Carbon dioxide may be absorbed into the blood stream at a rate of 100 ml/minute without adverse effect, but at absorption rates above this level hypercarbia may develop. This can lead to a fall in the blood pH, tachycardia and cardiac arrythmia or arrest. These undesirable side effects can be avoided by intubating and hyperventilating the patient during anaesthesia and monitoring the intra-abdominal pressure to ensure that it stays below 15 mmHg. Above this level the absorption rate is higher and there is an increased risk of side effects.

In the presence of water vapour in the peritoneal cavity, CO_2 forms carbonic acid (H_2CO_3) which is highly irritant and painful. Diaphragmatic irritation with H_2CO_3 is the source of referred shoulder pain experienced by many patients. The unwary physician may treat such pain inappropriately with anti-coagulants which, in the early post-operative period, may produce unwelcome complications. Fortunately, CO_2 embolism is a rare complication, but can be rapidly lethal. It has been reported in 1 : 10 000 to 1 : 60 000 cases but is probably under-diagnosed and under-reported because of the high solubility of CO_2 in blood. Early diagnosis may be made by the detection by auscultation of a precordial 'mill wheel' murmur or by Doppler ultrasonic monitoring during the operation.

Cardiac arrest may occur with the use of CO_2 and may be precipitated by overdistension, vasovagal reflex, a steep Trendelenburg position, the type of pre-medication or anaesthetic, hypoventilation or hypercarbia. The commonest cause, however, is gas embolism which is more likely to occur when the intra-abdominal gas pressure is higher than the systemic venous pressure. Hence the absolute necessity of closely monitoring the intra-abdominal pressure during gas insufflation and never exceeding 15 mmHg.

Nitrous Oxide

Nitrous oxide is less soluble in blood or body fluids than CO_2 but is about 14 times more soluble than air. It does not cause circulatory changes although there may be transient tachycardia during insufflation. The risk of gas embolism appears to be similar to that of CO_2.

Although N_2O is not flammable, it does support combustion. If methane or hydrogen gas should escape into the peritoneal cavity as a result of inadvertent puncture of bowel by a trocar or needle, a potentially explosive mixture of gases is produced which can cause a fatal accident if a high frequency electric current is used.

Nitrous oxide causes less pain than CO_2 and therefore has been preferred by gastro-enterologists when laparoscopy is performed under local anaesthesia.

Pneumoflator

A large number of commercially produced gas insufflation systems are available. There are two basic types: mechanical and electronic.

Mechanical pneumoflator

A mechanically controlled pneumoflator is adequate for diagnostic laparoscopy and for performing simple operations (Fig. 2.1). It will allow insufflation during filling of the abdomen at a rate of 1 l/minute which can then be increased to 3 l/minute for rapid filling under visual control. There may be significant loss of gas which must be replaced when performing more complex procedures during which it is necessary to change instruments frequently and to aspirate the plumes caused by laser or electrocoagulation or to remove fluid after peritoneal lavage. In these circumstances the mechanical pneumoflator is not sufficiently responsive and an electronic pneumoflator should be used.

Electronic pneumoflator

It is unsafe for the surgeon to have to check the function of the insufflation apparatus, the amount of abdominal distension and the

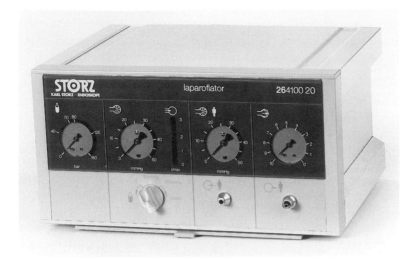

Fig. 2.1 Mechanically controlled pneumoflator.

intra-peritoneal pressure at the same time as a complicated laparo-scopic operation is being performed. The electronic pneumoflator (Fig. 2.2) is fully automatic and simultaneously measures the intra-abdominal and insufflation pressures which can be preset to cut out at a selected level. The amount of gas lost is determined electronically by the apparatus and automatically replaced at a rate of up to 6 l/minute so surgeons may be confident that the pneumoperiton-

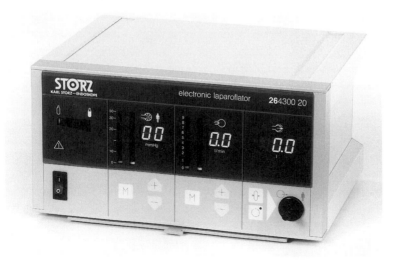

Fig. 2.2 Electronic pneumoflator.

eum is being maintained safely while they concentrate on the operation. Nothing is more frustrating and potentially dangerous than to lose the view at a crucial moment in a complex operation. The electronic pneumoflator prevents this occurrence.

Insufflating needle

The creation of the pneumoperitoneum may be effected through an insufflating needle. The most common needle in use is the Veress' needle which is spring-loaded and available in three lengths from 7 to 15 cm. The shortest is suitable for all but the very obese patient (Fig. 2.3). The instrument has a round-ended sheath. The needle has a blunt trocar which protrudes beyond the needle tip. The spring loading allows the blunt trocar to retract as the needle is inserted through the abdominal wall but to be extruded as soon as the peritoneal cavity is entered. This protects the viscera from perforation by the sharp needle tip.

A number of disposable needles are available which have the advantage of always being sharp but the disadvantage of being more expensive.

Occasionally, the abdominal wall is very thick or scarred. In such cases a special Veress' needle equipped with a collar to prevent too deep penetration can be introduced through the posterior vaginal fornix.

Primary trocar and cannula

Once the pneumoperitoneum has been produced, the next step is to introduce the telescope. The basic equipment for this is the primary

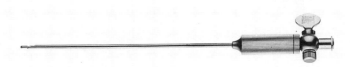

Fig. 2.3 Veress' needle.

trocar and cannula. The diameter of the trocar and cannula should correspond to the diameter of the telescope. The cannula should be equipped with a proximally sited valve to prevent gas leakage and a gas inflow channel with a tap. The distal opening may be straight or oblique; the latter may make insertion easier (Fig. 2.4).

The trocar may be solid or hollow. The advantage of the hollow trocar is that it signals entry into the peritoneal cavity by permitting some gas to escape. The distal tip of the trocar must be sharp. A blunt trocar requires more effort to insert; this poses a greater hazard of sudden deep penetration and resultant damage to a viscus.

The tip of the trocar may be pyramidal or conical. The pyramidal trocar has three surfaces with relatively sharp edges between them. Thus it requires less force to insert, but the sharp edge is more likely to cut a blood vessel in the abdominal wall. The conical trocar requires more force but is less likely to damage a blood vessel.

Disposable trocars and cannulae are available and are increasing in popularity because they are always sharp and therefore the amount of force needed to insert them is predictable.

Detailed examination of the abdominal or pelvic organs requires that they be retracted. Although a Veress' needle can be used as a retractor, its narrow diameter carries some risk of inadvertent perforation of a viscus. Retraction is best performed with a blunt probe which is calibrated in centimetres to facilitate measurement. This probe can also be used to place adhesions on stretch prior to division.

Laparoscopes

The modern laparoscope is a rigid telescope with a rod lens system

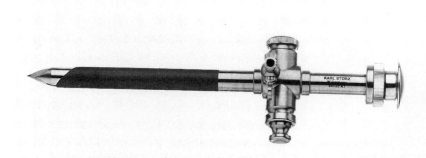

Fig. 2.4 Pyramidal trocar and cannula with an oblique distal opening.

which gives a bright image, excellent definition and a wide viewing angle.

Standard diagnostic laparoscopes vary from 5 to 11 mm in diameter. The 5 mm laparoscope gives an adequate view for inspection and simple operations such as sterilization, but the available light and field of vision is not satisfactory for the performance of more complex procedures or for the use of video.

The distal lens may be set at an angle of zero or 30°. The head on view provided by the 0° lens system makes orientation easier but, on occasion, fixity of the pelvic tissues by adhesions or endometriosis may hinder manipulation with ancillary instruments. In these circumstances the offset view provided by the 30° angle lens will allow the surgeon to inspect otherwise inaccessible tissues. In practice it is often a matter of personal preference which lens is used.

The operating laparoscope has an offset proximal lens and a channel through which ancillary instruments, and particularly laser fibres, can be inserted (Fig. 2.5). The proximal lens may be parallel or at an angle to the axis of the telescope. The advantage is that one less ancillary portal is required for the introduction of extra instruments. The telescope is larger and heavier, the viewing angle is narrower, and less light is transmitted. In addition it is not possible to separate the visual axis from the operating axis. In the opinion of many surgeons it is highly desirable that operating instruments can be introduced independently of the viewing system.

Instruments of small diameter are available for use in the paediatric patient. This is becoming more important as the general surgeons increase the use of diagnostic and operative laparoscopy for conditions such as appendicitis.

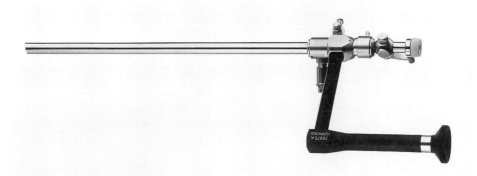

Fig. 2.5 Operating laparoscope with parallel proximal lens.

Light sources and cables

The standard 150 watt light source gives enough illumination for diagnostic laparoscopy. The performance of operative procedures and the use of video cameras require a more powerful light. A cold light fountain with a 250 watt halogen lamp is essential (Fig. 2.6).

The light must be transmitted from its source to the laparoscope by a fibreoptic or liquid filled cable. The liquid cable is more expensive but, because there are no fibreoptic light bundles and no risk of them breaking, the light is brighter and the cable does not deteriorate with use.

Video systems

As the scope of laparoscopy increases to involve more precise inspection and more complex operations, so the need to be able to demonstrate lesions and to operate in comfort and with assistance becomes necessary. The modern laparoscopist should be trained in video-laparoscopy which allows the surgeon to work in a comfortable standing position watching the video screen instead of crouching over the telescope. All the instruments can be reached with ease, which may be impossible if the surgeon is viewing through the lens. The assistant can follow the operation. It is also easier and safer to train and supervise junior staff.

The modern silicon chip camera weighs as little as 130 g and has a zoom lens with automatic colour setting and a high speed shutter to eliminate over-exposure (Fig. 2.7). The light source, video recorder

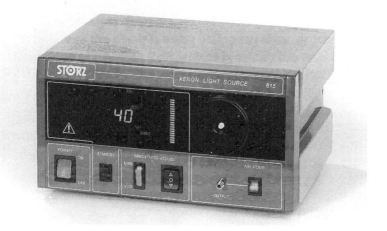

Fig. 2.6 Xenon Video Cold Light Fountain 615.

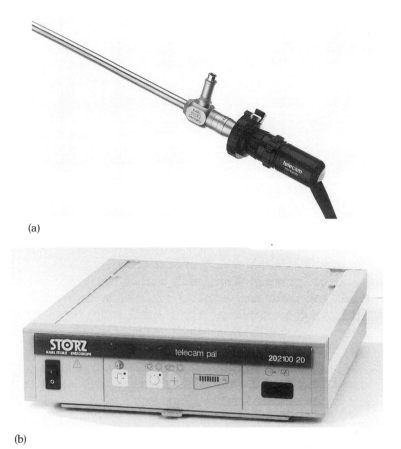

(a)

(b)

Fig. 2.7 (a) Silicone chip camera on diagnostic laparoscope; (b) camera control unit.

and pneumoflator may all be accommodated on a mobile endoscopy trolley making operating room management more efficient.

Ancillary instruments

A wide range of instruments has been developed to allow a large variety of operations of increasing complexity to be performed laparoscopically.

Forceps

A number of forceps are available. It is possible, and indeed preferable, to use a relatively small number. The surgeon should have two or three forceps, one or two with atraumatic blades and another with teeth for stronger traction (Fig. 2.8).

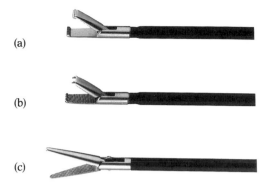

(a)

(b)

(c)

Fig. 2.8 Laparoscopic
forceps: (a) blunt ended
atraumatic forceps;
(b) toothed forceps;
(c) sharp ended
atraumatic forceps.

Forceps with scissor grips are easily applied. The blades of forceps with spring-loaded grips tend to withdraw into the shaft of the instrument during application. The forceps should be designed to give the surgeon the option of working free hand as well as having a locking device for firmer traction.

Scissors

Scissors which will pass through a 5.5 mm cannula are fine enough to perform accurate dissection. Microscissors can be used for adhesiolysis close to the fimbriae if more delicate dissection is required. Hook scissors are designed to pull the tissues into the cutting blades. Straight self-sharpening scissors allow more accurate incision of tissues. It is important that one of the scissor blades is fixed as this allows the scissors to be used to exert gentle traction before cutting (Fig. 2.9).

Larger scissors with a diameter of 11 mm may occasionally be needed to divide tough tissues or to morcellate a lesion prior to removal through a cannula. Similar 11 mm forceps may also be necessary to provide strong traction (Fig. 2.10).

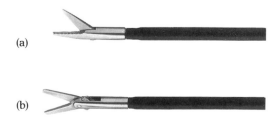

(a)

(b)

Fig. 2.9 Laparoscopic
scissors: (a) scissors
with one fixed blade;
(b) scissors with two
mobile blades.

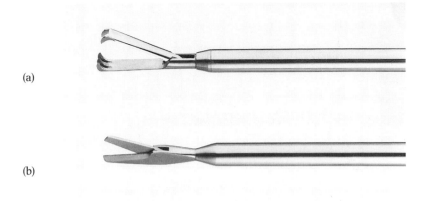

(a)

(b)

Fig. 2.10 Eleven mm instruments: (a) claw forceps; (b) scissors.

Electrosurgical instruments

The ability to coagulate tissues to prevent or control bleeding is one of the prerequisites of any surgical procedure. Facility to use both monopolar and bipolar current is essential. Some laparoscopists prefer thermocoagulation on the grounds of safety and, possibly, less tissue destruction.

Electrosurgical units are machines which produce an alternating electrical current at a frequency which will not stimulate neuromuscular activity. Direct current flows in one direction only, but alternating current flows to and fro in both directions, producing a sinusoidal wave form (Fig. 2.11). A pure cutting current is a simple sinusoidal wave form. Because it is continuous it does not need to be at high power. If the point of application is small, the power setting may be low. Thus a cutting current applied through a microneedle provides an instrument capable of incising tissues with safety because the power at the point of impact is low.

The current must return to the electrosurgical unit to complete the electrical circuit. When a monopolar current is used, the current passes back through a return plate which should be placed as close as possible to the operation site. It is important that the return plate has a large surface area. This ensures that the power density at that point is low and that there is no danger of a skin burn. Bipolar current is applied to the tissues through the blades of forceps, one blade of which acts as the positive electrode and the other as the negative. The electric current thus passes from one blade to the other without spread of current through the body tissues.

Coagulation of tissues may be produced by a damped wave form

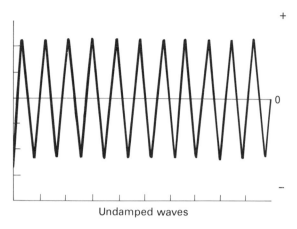

Fig. 2.11 Pure or cutting current.

which produces an intermittent high voltage current (Fig. 2.12). Thus there may be a high voltage within the tissues for an instant. If this high voltage is used with a monopolar current the electric current may jump to nearby structures, with risk of inadvertent burns.

The instruments used for electrosurgery include monopolar microneedles, hooks, forceps and scissors and bipolar forceps of varying breadth. The fine bipolar forceps are generally more useful (Figs. 2.13 and 2.14).

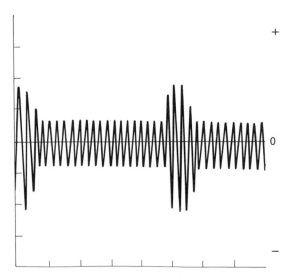

Fig. 2.12 Combined or blended waves give cutting-coagulation effect.

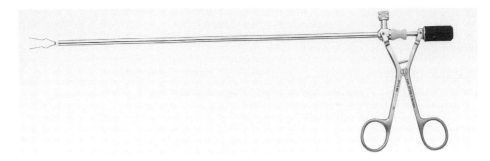

Fig. 2.13 Fine bipolar forceps.

Laser

The carbon dioxide (CO_2) laser provides a precise method of tissue incision which produces little thermal damage. It produces vaporization of tissues to a depth of 0.2–0.4 mm, which allows it to be used safely close to vital structures. The major limitations of the CO_2 laser are that it cannot be used in a fluid medium and it has poor coagulating properties. The laser beam may be passed through the laparoscope using a coupling device or through a secondary cannula.

The Nd : YAG, Argon and KTP lasers can be passed down flexible fibres and are easier to align; they produce better coagulation and are effective in a fluid medium. They produce deeper vaporization. The Nα : YAG laser penetrates 4–6 mm which is too deep to use safely near vital structures.

(a)

(b)

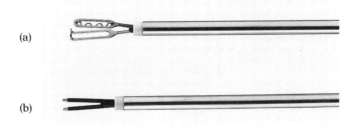

Fig. 2.14 Bipolar forceps: (a) bipolar grasping forceps; (b) bipolar micro forceps.

Sutures and ligatures

Sutures

The value of sutures in some circumstances is debatable whilst in others, sutures are essential. These issues will be discussed in detail in Chapter 4

Two suturing techniques are used in laparoscopic surgery. In the first the knot is tied using instruments within the abdomen. In the second the suture is tied extra-corporeally. Ancillary equipment for suturing should include:

1 Needle holders which are fine enough to hold the smallest needles and shaped to assist tying the knot.
2 Grasping forceps to catch the needle as it is inserted and to assist intra-abdominal knot tying.
3 A knot pusher with which to tighten knots tied outside the abdomen.
4 Short straight or ski needles which can be inserted into the abdomen through a 5 mm cannula.

Ligatures

Ligatures are most easily applied by using a prepacked modified Roeder loop introduced through the standard 5 mm cannula with a special applicator.

Clips and staples

Modifications of the Weck haemoclip are invaluable for prevention and control of bleeding. The clips may be absorbable or non-absorbable and may be applied singly or in multiples with disposable or re-usable applicators.

Instruments are now available which will apply up to three rows of staples on either side of the line where an incision is to be made. A blade contained within the instrument makes the incision. Control of both stapling and cutting is effected by means of a proximal pistol grip. Currently, these instruments are disposable and expensive.

Flushing and suction instruments

Irrigation with warm physiological fluids is an integral part of all but the simplest laparoscopic operations. Suction capability is required to remove the irrigation fluid, blood, debris and smoke resulting from

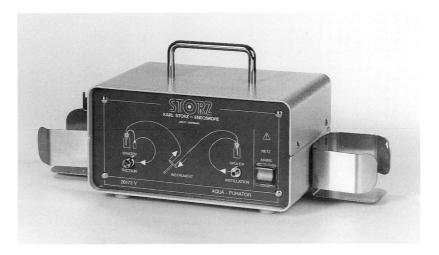

Fig. 2.15 Automatic irrigation pump.

the use of intra-abdominal energy sources. Both functions can be performed conveniently by using a combined irrigation and suction cannula connected to an automatic pump (Fig. 2.15). The system is controlled by a hand held mechanism. The cannula may be provided with a channel through which grasping forceps or electrodes may be inserted.

Needles

Needles with which cysts may be aspirated or haemostatic fluids injected should be available. The former should have a wide bore needle on the end of a suction cannula. A spinal needle for the injection of pitressin or adrenaline haemostatic solutions can be introduced directly through the abdominal wall.

Conclusion

There is a very wide choice of laparoscopic equipment. The ideal set has yet to be devised. This chapter provides a description of those pieces of equipment believed to be essential for the performance of effective diagnostic and operative laparoscopy.

3: Diagnostic Laparoscopy

Introduction

Diagnostic laparoscopy is indicated in any situation when inspection of the abdominal or pelvic organs will help to establish a diagnosis and to define subsequent management. Laparoscopy should be preceded by taking a full clinical history and performing a careful clinical examination. Pre-operative investigations should be performed as indicated and may include laboratory, radiological and sonar investigation. Laparoscopy is increasingly being used as a means of access to allow surgical procedures to be performed. Often an operation which starts as a diagnostic procedure may become an operative laparoscopy. These operative procedures will be discussed in subsequent chapters in this book.

Technique

Pre-operative check list

Before the patient is brought into the operating room, the surgeon must ensure that the insufflator is functioning and has an adequate supply of gas and that the electric generator, light source and video equipment are all in perfect working order. Once the patient has been anaesthetized and prepared, the surgeon should also be assured that all the equipment necessary for the performance of the operation is present and functioning. Nothing is more frustrating than to discover that the light cable is not compatible with the light post on the telescope or that incorrect electrical leads have been provided.

Anaesthesia

A general anaesthetic with muscle relaxation, endotracheal intubation and assisted respiration should be administered. Relaxation of the abdominal muscles greatly facilitates the introduction and manipulation of the instruments. Laparoscopy with carbon dioxide (CO_2) carries a risk of hypercarbia. Absorption of CO_2 and splinting of the diaphragm both by the pressure of the pneumoperitoneum and the necessity of placing the patient in the Trendelenburg position aggravate this risk. It is for this reason that endotracheal intubation and assisted respiration, continuous monitoring of the heart rate, blood pressure and blood gases are mandatory.

Positioning of the patient

The operating table should be capable of tilting in both axes. Normally, diagnostic laparoscopy only requires a 15° Trendelenburg tilt but a steeper angle may be used for some operative procedures. Lateral tilting helps to expose the pelvic side walls and, with modern laparoscopic surgery including operations on the ureters, kidneys and spleen, as well as the gall bladder and pelvic organs, the need for a lateral tilt becomes important. When a steeper angle is used for operative laparoscopy it is essential to have a non-slip mattress to prevent the patient moving cephalad on the table.

The patient should be placed in the supine position with the legs abducted and supported in a modified lithotomy position. Diagnostic laparoscopy may be performed with the legs flexed to 45° but the legs should be almost flat during laparoscopic pelvic surgery to allow the full range of movements of instruments such as scissors and forceps (Fig. 3.1). The patient's buttocks should protrude over the edge of the table to allow the uterus to be manipulated by an intra-uterine cannula.

Great care must be taken. The anaesthetized patient is helpless and very vulnerable to compression injuries of the brachial plexus,

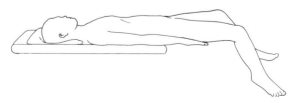

Fig. 3.1 Position of the patient on the operating table.

nerves of the legs and leg veins. Carelessly placed hands can be trapped in moving parts of the operating table. If any part of the patient is in contact with a metal object she will be at risk of electrosurgical burns at this point.

Preparation for laparoscopy

The abdominal wall should be cleansed with an antiseptic solution paying special attention to the umbilicus. At the same time, an assistant should wash the vulva and vagina, catheterize the bladder and apply a tenaculum to the cervix and insert a uterine cannula. This cannula should be sufficiently long to reach the uterine fundus to allow effective manipulation of the uterus and should have the capability for performing chromopertubation.

Insertion of Veress' needle

The surgeon should first check that the Veress' needle is patent and its spring mechanism is functioning. It should be connected to the pneumoflator and the gas turned on so that the basal pressure in the system can be noted. Insufflation pressure should not rise more than 5–10 mmHg above this pressure. The site of insertion must be chosen. The optimum site is deep in the umbilicus because:

1 The abdominal wall is thinnest in that position and is made up of skin, fascia and peritoneum with no intervening fat. Thus, even in obese patients, a pneumoperitoneum can be produced with a 7 cm needle.

2 The peritoneum is closely applied to the underlying fascia and does not peel off as it does in other sites. This decreases the possibility of extra-peritoneal insufflation of gas occurring.

3 The incision is cosmetic and is often invisible within 2–3 weeks whereas an incision below the umbilicus always leaves a permanent scar.

It may be necessary to choose an alternative site if adhesions are suspected in, for instance, the presence of a vertical sub-umbilical scar. Other possible sites are lateral to the umbilicus at the same level, supra-pubically in the mid-line or, possibly better, in the left hypochondrium or posterior vaginal fornix.

The technique of needle insertion through the umbilicus is as follows:

1 A small incision should be made in the depth of the umbilicus.

2 The abdominal wall should be held up with the free hand to prevent damage to underlying viscera and deep vessels (Fig. 3.2). If

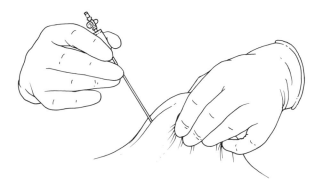

Fig. 3.2 Holding abdominal wall to insert Veress' needle.

the patient is very obese it may be difficult to grip the fat abdominal wall securely. In this case an assistant may help by pressing the abdomen on either side of the umbilicus to make it prominent while the surgeon grasps the wall with the full span of the hand. It is never necessary to lift the abdominal wall with a towel clip or sutures, both of which will cause unnecessary post-operative pain.

3 The needle should be held by the milled ring in such a way that the blunt inner obturator can move freely. It is inserted into the incision. The hub of the needle will be seen to move backwards as the resistance of the abdominal wall is met and will move rapidly forwards accompanied by an audible click as it pierces the fascia and again as it enters the peritoneal cavity. The insertion should always be at right angles to the surface and at 45° to the horizontal to prevent the needle point passing into the fat or muscle layers below the umbilicus and producing an extra-peritoneal insufflation of gas or injuring a major vessel.

4 The position of the needle must now be checked by the aspiration test. This may be performed in two ways:

(a) A 20 ml syringe is attached to the needle and the plunger withdrawn to make sure that the needle tip is not in the bowel or a major vessel. If no fluid or gas is obtained by this aspiration it is safe to inject 20 ml of air into the peritoneal cavity. If the needle tip is correctly situated, the air will be dispersed between loops of bowel and, when the aspiration is repeated, no air will be withdrawn (Fig. 3.3). If the needle is in the abdominal wall or in an adhesion, the air will not have been dispersed and will be aspirated back into the syringe. The needle must be resited if any of these occur.

(b) A 20 ml syringe filled with normal saline is used for the initial aspiration and will be stained brown or red if the tip is in the bowel or a vessel. The saline is then injected and the aspiration

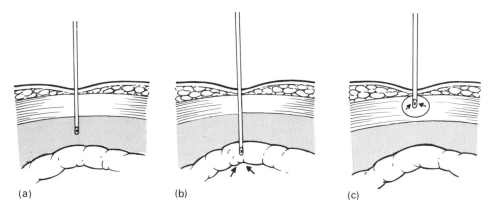

(a)   (b)   (c)

Fig. 3.3 (a) Needle tip correctly placed; (b) needle in a loop of bowel; (c) in the abdominal wall.

repeated (Fig. 3.4). Again, nothing will be withdrawn if the tip is correctly sited but, if it is in the abdominal wall, a vessel or a viscus, the aspirate will be clear, red or brown.

5 When the tip of the needle has been confirmed to be correctly situated in the peritoneal cavity, the pneumoperitoneum may be induced by insufflating CO_2 initially at 1 l/minute and, when free flow is established and the intra-abdominal pressure is below 15 mmHg, the rate may be increased to 2 l/minute. Higher flow rates should only be used under direct visual control. The total volume used will depend on the build of the patient and the procedure to be

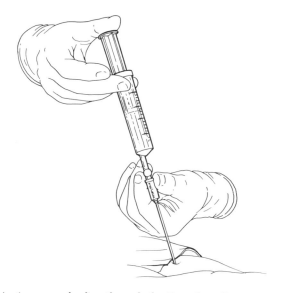

Fig. 3.4 Injecting normal saline through the Veress' needle.

performed. Diagnostic laparoscopy or tubal sterilization of a slim patient will require only 0.5–1.5 l whereas an obese patient requiring detailed examination or laparoscopic surgery may need 3–4 l of gas.

6 When the pneumoperitoneum is established, the presence of sufficient intra-abdominal space into which the laparoscope can be inserted safely should be confirmed by the sounding test. A 5 cm needle is attached to a 20 ml syringe and inserted through the abdominal wall below the umbilicus. Gas may be aspirated if there is free space but no gas will be withdrawn if the needle tip is in an adhesion. In this case the limits of the pneumoperitoneum may be mapped out by exploring the space in several directions and its depth may also be estimated by inserting the needle deeper. Thus a safe space into which to insert the primary trocar and cannula may be defined (Fig. 3.5).

If there are adhesions or if the patient is exceptionally obese, the pneumoperitoneum may be inserted through the posterior vaginal fornix. This is performed as follows:

1 The cervix should be exposed with a speculum, grasped with a tenaculum and displaced forwards to exert tension on the uterosacral ligaments and stretch the floor of the pouch of Douglas.

2 The needle may then be inserted in the mid-line, remembering that the depth of the floor of the pouch is only about 0.5 cm. The

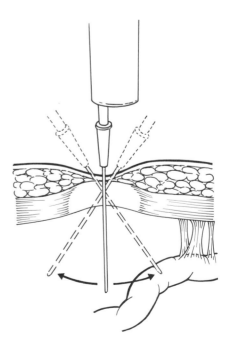

Fig. 3.5 Needle explores the pneumoperitoneum to detect adhesion.

aspiration test is then performed to ensure that the tip is free in the peritoneal cavity and the pneumoperitoneum induced.

3 The sounding test should then be performed as above to define a safe abdominal site for insertion of the laparoscope trocar and cannula.

Insertion of primary trocar and cannula

The primary trocar and cannula through which the laparoscope is introduced must now be inserted. A vertical incision is made through the skin from the small Veress' needle incision vertically towards the lower border of the umbilicus. The length of the incision will depend on the diameter of the laparoscope. The trocar and cannula is then held firmly with the flattened proximal end of the trocar in the heel of the hand (Fig. 3.6). During insertion the upper abdominal wall should be compressed by the free hand to make the lower abdomen tense and give a firm platform against which to insert the trocar and cannula. The trocar should be advanced along a zig-zag path to prevent incisional hernia and the extended fore-finger should act as a guard to prevent sudden deep insertion.

Insertion of laparoscope

The choice of laparoscope for diagnostic purposes is debatable. A 5 mm telescope may be inserted through the umbilicus without leaving any scar and may be satisfactory for simple examination of the pelvis. However, a larger telescope is preferable if video is used, as the available light allows a more detailed examination. In

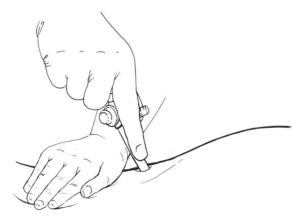

Fig. 3.6 Insertion of the primary trocar and cannula.

addition, if operative laparoscopy becomes necessary, the smaller telescope does not give sufficient light or field of vision.

When the trocar has been inserted and gas heard to escape through the cannula which confirms the tip is in the peritoneal cavity, a warmed telescope to which a camera has been attached may be introduced into the cannula and advanced under direct vision into the peritoneal cavity.

Insertion of secondary trocars and cannulae

During laparoscopy it may be necessary to insert second or third portals, the sites of which include:
1 The midline about 4 cm above the pubic symphysis. If the insertion is too low it may be difficult to reach the pouch of Douglas, especially if the uterus is retroverted. A lower insertion may put the bladder at risk. It is helpful to depress the abdominal wall with a finger at the site of the planned insertion, while watching with the laparoscope. This identifies its relationship to underlying organs and prevents inadvertent perforation of a viscus.
2 Within the 'safety triangle' which is formed by the umbilicus at its apex, the two obliterated umbilical arteries laterally and the pubic symphysis as its base. Instruments inserted within this area will rarely damage the deep inferior epigastric arteries, which may be seen by transillumination of the abdominal wall in thin patients. They may also be observed lateral to the obliterated umbilical artery through the laparoscope.
3 If these sites are inappropriate or if there are adhesions making them unsafe, the secondary portal may be inserted lateral to the rectus abdominis on either side.

The instruments should always be angled towards the pouch of Douglas with the uterus held in anteversion to allow space to develop behind it, into which the trocar may be safely inserted. Their entry should always be under direct laparoscopic observation.

Systematic inspection of the abdominal and pelvic organs

It is important that the inspection of the abdominal and pelvic organs is performed in a thorough and systematic manner.

The upper abdomen

The upper abdominal organs should be inspected in detail first

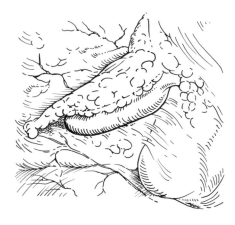

Fig. 3.7 Caecum and appendix.

before concentrating on the gynaecological examination. Following insertion of the laparoscope, the telescope should be rotated and the caecum and appendix examined using a probe or forceps to retract the caecum and expose the full length of the appendix (Fig. 3.7). The ascending colon is examined as far as the hepatic flexure. The presence of adhesions may indicate previous appendicular or gall bladder disease. It may be necessary to alter the Trendelenburg tilt to obtain a good view of the upper abdominal organs. The right lobe of the liver and the gall bladder should now be inspected and sub-diaphragmatic adhesions (Fitzhugh–Curtis syndrome) sought (Fig. 3.8). The telescope should be partially withdrawn to negotiate the ligamentum falciparum, and the left lobe of liver, anterior surface of the stomach and the spleen inspected. The examination of the upper abdomen is completed by further rotating the telescope to inspect the descending colon, using the forceps or probe to palpate the consistency of the bowel if diverticular disease is suspected. In this case the usual soft, mobile bowel may be more firm and less mobile. The general examination is completed by observing the

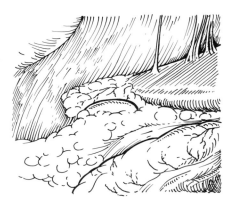

Fig. 3.8 Sub-diaphragmatic adhesions.

sigmoid colon, looking especially for evidence of diverticular disease, which may be suspected by the presence of adhesions and an altered consistency of the colon.

The pelvic organs

When the inspection of the upper abdomen is complete, attention should be given to the pelvic organs which should also be examined in a systematic manner. It is good practice to start with the uterus and then proceed from the anterior cul-de-sac in a clockwise direction round the pelvis to ensure that a full examination has been made.

1 *The uterus.* The size, position, shape and mobility of the uterus should all be noted (Fig. 3.9). Enlargement of the uterus may suggest intra-mural fibroids or adenomyosis, the differential diagnosis depending on the symmetry of the organ. Evidence of partial or complete failure of fusion of the Müllerian ducts may be relevent to recurrent abortion, and adhesions to other organs should also be noted.

2 *The anterior cul-de-sac.* The surface of the bladder is a frequent site of endometriosis and occasionally the bladder may be adherent to the anterior surface of the uterus as a result of endometriosis or previous surgery. After examining the right round ligament, the inspection should continue with evaluation of:

3 *The right fallopian tube.* The tube should be inspected throughout its length by lifting it with a probe or forceps. It is impossible to examine the tube and ovary fully without using a second instrument. The isthmic segment of the tube should be inspected for evidence of

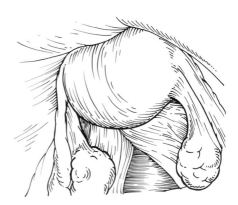

Fig. 3.9 Panoramic view of normal uterus tubes and ovaries.

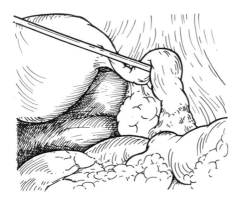

Fig. 3.10 Lifting the tube to visualize its full length.

swelling which could suggest salpingitis isthmica nodosa or endometriosis. In the former the swelling is usually uniform and, following chromopertubation, the sub-peritoneal blue blebs of methylene
blue are characteristic. The examination should continue with the
surgeon noting the diameter and thickness of the wall, and mobility
of the ampulla (Fig. 3.10). Distal tubal obstruction, peritubal adhesions, pseudohydrosalpinx which is seen on the antimesenteric wall
about 1 cm proximal to the fimbriae and, finally, the fimbriae
themselves, should all be observed and the findings noted.

4 *The right ovary.* The next structure to be seen is the right ovary,
which must be examined with the help of a probe or forceps so that
both sides may be seen. The size of the ovary should be noted.
Evidence of ovarian activity such as follicular or luteal cyst formation
should be correlated with the time in the menstrual cycle (Fig. 3.11).
Signs of endometriosis and peri-ovarian adhesions resulting from
endometriosis or infection may all be seen only after turning the
ovary over to enable its lateral aspect to be inspected.

5 *The right broad ligament.* After examining the right ovary, evidence
of endometriosis should be sought, especially in the ovarian fossa.

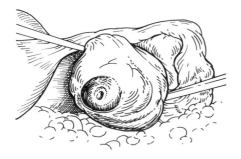

Fig. 3.11 The stigma seen soon
after ovulation.

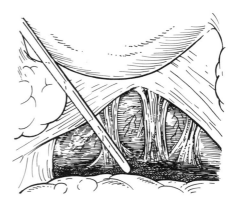

Fig. 3.12 Aspirating fluid from the pouch of Douglas.

Peritoneal defects (Allan Masters' syndrome) often have small deposits of endometriosis deep in the defect.

6 *The right utero-sacral ligament and the pouch of Douglas.* Finally, on the right side, the utero-sacral ligament and the floor of the pouch of Douglas should be inspected in detail. The Trendelenburg tilt may have to be increased to obtain a clear view of the floor of the pouch and it is often necessary to aspirate free fluid to be able to see all of the peritoneal surface (Fig. 3.12). Once again, these are common sites for endometriosis and, especially, deep endometriomas causing nodules in the ligaments or adhesions deep in the pouch should be sought. On occasion there may be no overt evidence of pelvic endometriosis and superficially the peritoneum, tube and ovary may appear to be healthy. When an attempt is made to mobilize the ovary with a probe it will be noted to be firmly adherent to the ovarian fossa. If the ovary is dissected free, evidence of endometriosis will invariably be noted in the ovarian fossa. The finding of two ovaries which are adherent in the mid-line, the so-called 'kissing ovaries', is pathognomonic of endometriosis.

7 *The left side of the pelvis.* The examination should now continue round the left side of the pelvis in reverse order, inspecting the broad ligament, ovary, tube and the left round ligament before coming back to the anterior cul-de-sac. Examination of the left tube may be more difficult because common but normal adhesions of the sigmoid colon to the left pelvic side wall frequently obscure the left tube, which must be lifted out of the pelvis to allow full inspection.

Infertility cases

Finally, in cases of infertility, inspection includes the following:

Chromopertubation

Once the pelvis has been thoroughly inspected, tubal patency may be tested. Dilute methylene blue (1 : 20 solution) should be injected through the cervical cannula and its passage along each fallopian tube followed. The passage of dye is usually preceded by bubbles of gas coming through the fimbriae. Normally, the fimbriae are flattened by the pressure of the pneumoperitoneum. They may best be seen if the pelvis is filled with Ringer lactate solution so that the terminal tube floats in the fluid, making peri-fimbrial adhesions much more obvious.

Salpingoscopy

More detailed examination of the tubal mucosa (salpingoscopy) should be performed in any patient with evidence of peri-tubal disease, tubal phimosis or distal tubal blockage. Its use may also be of value in cases of previous pelvic inflammatory disease or in patients who have had an ectopic pregnancy in the contra-lateral tube.

In salpingoscopy a rigid 3 mm telescope is passed along the channel of an operating laparoscope into the abdominal tubal ostium to inspect the ampullary mucosa. The instruments consist of:

1 A 10 mm or 11 mm operating laparoscope.

2 A sheath which fits into the operating channel and through which the salpingoscope will be passed. The sheath has a side aperture with a stopcock to allow introduction of an infusion of saline.

3 An obturator with a conical tip to aid introduction of the sheath into the tubal ostium. This is removed and replaced by:

4 A 3 mm telescope which is passed through the sheath after it has been inserted into the tube. The salpingoscope can move freely forwards and backwards to explore the full length of the ampulla. The telescope may have a lens mechanism to allow magnification and permit more detailed examination of the vasculature of the mucosal folds (Fig. 3.13).

5 A saline infusion with which to distend the ampulla to permit visualization. The infusion should be at a height of 1 m above the patient's body.

6 A pair of tube-holding forceps with which the tube is manipulated and grasped over the cannula to form a water-tight seal which allows tubal distension.

Prior to introducing the salpingoscope the tube must be aligned with the laparoscope by gentle manipulation with the forceps. Adhesions may have to be divided and, if there is distal tubal

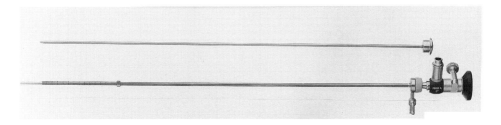

Fig. 3.13 Salpingoscope: obturator (top); salpingoscope within its protective sheath (botttom).

blockage, salpingostomy may have to be performed with an electrical micro-needle or laser. In this case only a very small opening is made until the tubal mucosa has been inspected.

The technique of salpingoscopy is as follows:

1 The uterus is first anteverted with an intra-uterine cannula. Tube-holding forceps are introduced through a secondary portal and the ovarian ligament grasped. The ovary and tube can then be lifted. The uterus is retroverted, rotated and the fundus displaced laterally into the ovarian fossa. This allows the tube and ovary to lie on the anterior surface of the uterus, which may be used as an 'internal operating table' on which the organs to be inspected lie (Fig. 3.14).

2 The tube is manipulated with the forceps until the fimbriae and abdominal ostium are in line with the laparoscope (Fig. 3.15).

3 The sheath with its obturator are advanced out of the operating channel into the tubal ostium, which may usually be found near the anti-mesenteric border of the fimbriae. The fallopian tube may be gently drawn on to the cannula by the forceps. The position of the sheath within the tube may be confirmed by opening the stopcock and watching the ampulla distend with the saline infusion.

4 The obturator is then withdrawn and replaced with the salpingo-

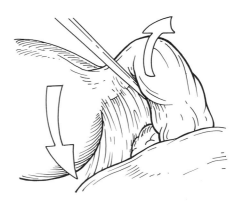

Fig. 3.14 Elevating the adnexae whilst retroverting and rotating the uterus.

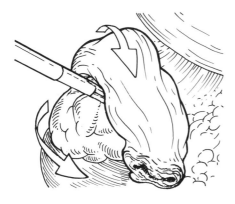

Fig. 3.15 The adnexae lying on the anterior surface of the uterus allowing the fimbrial opening to be seen.

scope, the saline infusion commenced and the salpingoscope advanced under direct vision to inspect the tubal mucosa as far as the isthmo-ampullary junction.

Fold patterns. Five fold patterns have been described:
1 The normal ampulla should have 5–6 major mucosal folds, each about 4–6 mm in height arranged radially (Fig. 3.16). They run longitudinally along the ampulla until they flatten and merge into low minor folds at the isthmo-ampullary junction. Secondary folds arise from the sides of the major folds and move freely in the fluid distending medium. Between the major folds are several minor folds about 1 mm in height, which become about half that size as they enter the tubal isthmus. The minor folds then continue along the isthmic and intra-mural segments of the tube and may sometimes be seen hysteroscopically in the uterine tubal ostium.
2 In hydrosalpinx with minor to moderate tubal distension, the folds may be flattened and wider apart than normal. These will usually revert to normal when the pressure on them is relieved (Fig. 3.17).

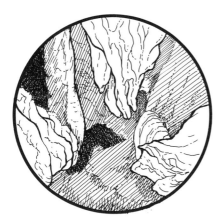

Fig. 3.16 Salpingoscopy grade 1: normal major mucosal folds with auxillary folds on their sides.

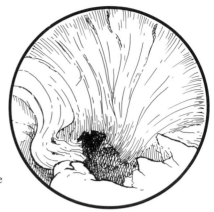

Fig. 3.17 Salpingoscopy grade 2: the major folds are flattened and wider apart.

The finding of grade 2 mucosal folds carries a good prognosis for tubal reconstructive surgery.

3 The mucosal folds are preserved but there are varying degrees of adhesion between the folds (Fig. 3.18). Fine focal adhesions appear to carry a relatively good prognosis but extensive adhesions, especially if they are tough and fibrous, or conglutination of the folds, suggest that there has been extensive mucosal cellular damage and carry a poor prognosis. Fine intra-tubal adhesions may be found in about 1.5% of tubes which look normal externally and are probably not significant.

4 Extensive mucosal lesions, with the folds densely adherent to each other (Fig. 3.19). There may also be stricture of the tube and formation of pseudospaces by complex intraluminal adhesions between the folds. Occasional pregnancies have been reported with these lesions but, in general, the prognosis is very poor.

5 The damage to the tubal wall and mucosa is extensive (Fig. 3.20).

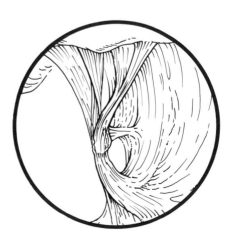

Fig. 3.18 Salpingoscopy grade 3: fibrous adhesions between the mucosal folds.

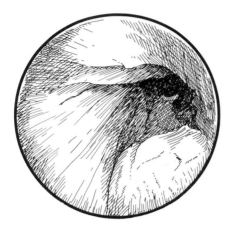

Fig. 3.19 Salpingoscopy grade 4: extensive mucosal adhesion with the folds densely adhered to each other.

There has been complete loss of fold pattern, the wall is rigid and the myosalpinx has been replaced by fibrous tissue. The outlook for pregnancy in tubes such as these is hopeless.

Salpingoscopy may thus be used as a decision maker to determine which patient with tubal infertility should be offered tubal reconstructive surgery and which should be referred for *in vitro* fertilization.

Skin closure

Once the diagnostic survey has been completed, the ancillary instruments and their cannulae are removed and the puncture sites inspected with the laparoscope to confirm that they are not bleeding. Finally, the gas is allowed to escape and the principal cannula is removed.

The small abdominal incisions should be closed with a non-

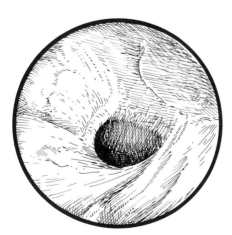

Fig. 3.20 Salpingoscopy grade 5: complete loss of fold pattern with a rigid fibrotic tubal wall.

absorbable suture which should be removed in 5–7 days. Alternatively, a subcutaneous absorbable suture may be used. It is important that skin dressings are removed on the first post-operative day because of the risk of infection.

Indications for diagnostic laparoscopy

Non-acute conditions

Diagnostic laparoscopy may be performed as a planned procedure for a number of non-acute conditions.

Infertility

This is one of the most common indications as the full investigation of infertility is never complete without actually visualizing the pelvic organs, although a preliminary hysterosalpingogram may be accepted as evidence of probable normality until reasonable time has been given for pregnancy to occur. The detailed examination of the abdomen and pelvis should always be performed, but in infertility patients several points should be noted:

1 Subdiaphragmatic adhesions may be the only evidence of a prior acute pelvic infection.

2 Developmental abnormalities of the uterus, and fibroids, especially if they are intramural or close to the fallopian tubes, should be noted.

3 The full length of the fallopian tubes should always be seen, and the proximal tube inspected for evidence of salpingitis isthmica nodosa or endometriosis. Ampullary swelling due to distal disease should be noted. The appearance of any hydrosalpinx and whether the tubal wall is thick or thin gives some prognostic information about the chance of surgical treatment being effective. Peritubal adhesions limiting tubal mobility and the appearance of the fimbriae and the patency of the fimbrial end of the tube are all important.

The fimbriae may be examined in greater detail by filling the pelvis with Ringer's lactate solution and examining the fimbriae under the surface of the fluid. The normal fimbriae will float in the fluid and any fine adhesions will be much more apparent.

4 The ovaries should be inspected in detail for signs of ovulatory activity and endometriosis. The size and evidence to support a diagnosis of polycystic ovarian disease should be sought.

Chronic pelvic pain

Systematic examination of the abdomen and pelvis may be necessary in cases of chronic pelvic pain, looking especially for evidence of infection, endometriosis or bowel disease including appendicitis. The bowel should be palpated with a probe to determine its consistency, which may be altered in diverticular disease when it may be less mobile, tending to move en masse when gently probed.

Suspected chronic pelvic inflammatory disease

The diagnosis of chronic pelvic inflammatory disease (PID) can only be made with certainty and its differentiation from endometriosis confirmed by laparoscopy. Frequently, there may be no history of an acute episode of pain but the patient may present with chronic discomfort or the diagnosis may be made during the routine investigation of infertility. It is always essential to inspect the liver and diaphragm for perihepatic adhesions.

Endometriosis

It is important to be aware of the appearance of early endometriosis, which may present as clear vesicles or an alteration of the pattern of the peritoneal blood vessels before progressing to red plaques and eventually to black plaques which are probably inactive. The sequelae of endometriosis or adhesion formation with resulting pain or infertility may be an indication for quite difficult and extensive laparoscopic surgery. Endometriosis deep in the pouch of Douglas may only be diagnosed by a combination of laparoscopy and digital vaginal and rectal examination to detect an endometrioma in the recto-vaginal septum.

Uterine abnormalities

Congenital uterine abnormalities may be associated with infertility or recurrent pregnancy loss. The appearance of the septate uterus with a dimple in a broad fundus is typical and it is important to exclude complete division of the horns of a bicornuate uterus before considering hysteroscopic resection of the septum. Other deformities such as unicornuate uterus or rudimentary horn should be noted, although there is no surgical treatment for them. It is probable that in the future newer imaging techniques may replace laparoscopy in the assessment of uterine abnormalities.

Laparoscopy is sometimes helpful in the assessment of fibroids, especially their relation to the intra-mural segment of the fallopian tube. However, high resolution transvaginal ultrasound has replaced laparoscopy in many such investigations.

Prior to tubal surgery

It is only justifiable to offer tubal reconstructive surgery if there is a reasonable prospect of success. A full evaluation of the tube, which can only be performed by laparoscopy and salpingoscopy, is a prerequisite to distal tubal surgery.

Acute conditions

Laparoscopy is an essential part of the investigation of many acute intra-abdominal conditions but should be combined with a full and detailed clinical history, a complete physical examination and judicious use of ultrasound and laboratory facilities. Frequently, laparoscopy may be used not only as a diagnostic tool but as a means of access to perform therapeutic surgery and thus avoid laparotomy. Even if laparoscopic surgery is not feasible, preliminary laparoscopy will help to plan the most effective incision and avoid the unsightly long vertical incision favoured by some general surgeons.

Frequently it is impossible to make a precise diagnosis in the presence of acute abdominal pain without recourse to laparoscopy. The presentation of acute PID, appendicitis, rupture or perforation of a viscus may be confusing and resolution of doubt may only be obtained by laparoscopy.

Acute pelvic inflammatory disease

Laparoscopy may be necessary to establish the diagnosis of PID and to differentiate it from appendicitis or an ectopic pregnancy. Occasionally, the tubes may not look obviously inflamed and in these cases culture of fluid from the pouch of Douglas may be unrewarding. Intra-luminal swabs and a search for sub-diaphragmatic adhesions may give the only clue to the diagnosis.

Ectopic pregnancy

Laparoscopy is becoming less important in the diagnosis of ectopic pregnancy with the advent of high resolution transvaginal ultrasonography and accurate estimation of β-HCG levels. However the surgical treatment of most ectopic pregnancies should be by a laparoscopic approach.

Torsion of a tube or ovary

Torsion of a viscus may be diagnosed by the history and with the use of ultrasound. The viability of the tube or ovary may only be ascertained by inspection and laparoscopy may often provide a means of treatment by untwisting the tube or ovary and, in the case of the ovary, shortening the ovarian ligament to prevent recurrence. Laparoscopy provides the means of removing the organ if it is infarcted.

Contra-indications to laparoscopy

Absolute contra-indications

Laparoscopy is absolutely contra-indicated in a number of conditions:
1 A large abdominal mass such as a fibroid or large ovarian cyst.
2 An irreducible external hernia because the increased intra-abdominal pressure may cause more loops of bowel to enter the hernial sac and make the condition worse.
3 Hypovolaemic shock, which should be corrected before any surgical procedure is undertaken. This is more important in laparoscopy where the added cardiac embarrassment produced by the pneumoperitoneum may be fatal.
4 Coincidental medical conditions such as cardio-respiratory failure, obstructive airways disease or a recent myocardial infarct.
5 An inexperienced surgeon or lack of proper facilities.

Relative contra-indications

Other conditions may be looked upon as relative contra-indications although their significance will depend to some degree on the general condition of the patient as well as the experience of the surgeon.
1 Multiple abdominal incisions may pose an increased risk and must be treated with respect. The patient should be forewarned of the risk. Application of the standard safety protocols should reduce this risk.
2 The mechanical problem posed by gross obesity may be dealt with by introducing the pneumoperitoneum through the floor of the

pouch of Douglas and using a long trocar and cannula to introduce the laparoscope.

3 Local skin infection may also necessitate a different site of insertion of instruments.

4 Generalized peritonitis, although many surgeons will now use the laparoscope to treat as well as diagnose the cause of peritonitis.

5 Intestinal obstruction or ileus, because of the danger of perforation of the bowel by the Veress' needle or a primary trocar before the abdomen has been inspected. The safety of laparoscopy in the presence of intestinal obstruction depends on the degree of bowel distension.

6 Coincidental medical conditions such as ischaemic heart disease, blood dyscrasia and coagulopathies.

4: Principles of Operative Laparoscopy

Introduction

Laparoscopic surgery is a natural extension of diagnostic laparo-scopy. The development of instruments to perform surgical oper-ations using the laparoscope to gain access to the abdominal cavity has revolutionized gynaecological practice. Mechanical and electrical instruments and lasers have all contributed to the advances of the past decade. Reliable methods of haemostasis make it safe to perform extensive surgery of the fallopian tubes, ovaries and uterus which hitherto was only considered possible by laparotomy. More ad-vanced operations including myomectomy, pelvic lymphadenectomy and hysterectomy have opened even wider possibilities to the gynae-cologist. The general surgeons, urologists and thoracic surgeons have also developed new techniques to replace the time-honoured laparotomy and thoracotomy. In experienced hands laparoscopic surgery can now replace laparotomy in up to 75% of cases, and the time has come when this form of surgery must be considered a standard technique in which all surgeons should be trained.

General principles of laparoscopic surgery

The safe performance of laparoscopic surgery demands that certain basic principles be observed meticulously.

1 There must always be a proper indication for the operation and the choice of laparoscopic surgery must be appropriate.

2 The patient should be under general anaesthesia with good relaxation, endotracheal intubation and controlled positive pressure ventilation.

3 Appropriate instruments must be readily available in the operating

room. These must be well maintained and in good working order.

4 There must be adequate assistance by staff who understand the principles of laparoscopic surgery.

5 There should be adequate space available in which to work. This is achieved by using an electronically controlled pneumoperitoneum apparatus and a steep Trendelenburg position. The bowels should be manipulated out of the pelvis and the bladder should be empty. The bowel should be prepared to ensure that it is empty and pre-operative antibiotics should be given in cases where there may be risk of bowel damage.

6 Gentle tissue handling is imperative at all times.

7 The surgeon must be able to recognize landmarks in the abdomen and pelvis. Prior to performing the surgery, the following should be identified if possible and the landmarks used to plan the best surgical approach. If they are hidden by adhesions they should be identified as soon as possible by dividing the adhesions.

  (a) Intra-abdominal structures if appropriate.
      Appendix and caecum
      Liver and gall bladder
      Stomach and small bowel
      Omentum and transverse colon, especially before and after extensive surgery.
  (b) Intra-pelvic structures:
      Obliterated umbilical arteries (safety triangle)
      Uterus, fallopian tubes and ovaries
      Bladder
      Ureter
      External iliac vessels
      Sigmoid colon and rectum
      Utero-sacral ligaments.
  (c) Retroperitoneal structures:
      Bifurcation of aorta and common iliac vessels,
      especially before and after extensive surgery.

8 Tissues must never be cut or burnt unless they can be seen clearly. If using monopolar electric current, the surgeon must ensure that the target tissue is not in contact with any other organ, or a burn may occur at the site of contact which may be outside the visual field.

9 The surgeon should be competent and trained in this form of surgery. Laparoscopic surgery has limitations. The surgeon should remain humble at all times and know when it is prudent to abandon the laparoscopic approach.

All laparoscopic surgery begins with a full and detailed examination of the abdomen and pelvis as described in Chapter 3. It is important to be aware of the normal anatomy of the pelvis and at all times to know which organs are likely to lie close to or behind the operation site. Adhesiolysis close to the bowel is potentially dangerous and the use of electricity or laser energy on tissues overlying the ureter may lead to disastrous complications. Care and a high level of awareness are necessary at all times.

The majority of laparoscopists use a 0° 10–11 mm diagnostic laparoscope and insert ancillary instruments through separate portals. Some use an operating laparoscope which has a channel for instruments such as forceps or laser, but these laparoscopes are heavier and have a narrower field of vision which can make surgery more difficult.

Specific principles of laparoscopic surgery

Position of the surgeon

A right-handed surgeon should usually stand on the patient's left (Fig. 4.1). The laparoscope is inserted through the umbilicus and, for pelvic surgery, ancillary instruments lower in the abdomen. It is not possible to perform complex laparoscopic surgery while viewing through the lens. It is always necessary to use closed circuit television (CCTV) and work viewing the video screen. Two techniques are commonly used:

1 The surgeon holds the laparoscope and camera in the right hand. An assistant steadies the tissues with grasping forceps and the surgeon holds the active instrument (scissors, electrosurgical instrument or laser) in the left hand (Fig. 4.2).

2 The assistant holds the laparoscope and camera and the surgeon holds both ancillary instruments.

It is a matter of personal preference which technique is used. In practice, a mixture of both gives the best results.

Access to the pelvis

It is always necessary to obtain a clear view of the pelvic organs before any laparoscopic surgery is performed. The appearances may differ from those seen during laparotomy because of the abdominal distension, which alters relationships to some degree. The laparoscope is normally inserted through the umbilicus, although some-

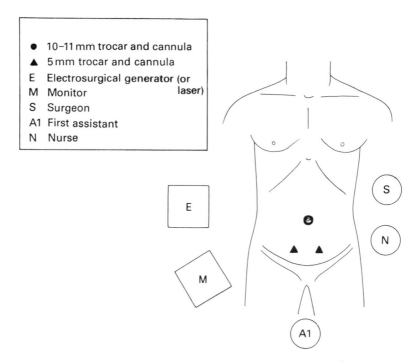

● 10–11 mm trocar and cannula
▲ 5 mm trocar and cannula
E Electrosurgical generator (or laser)
M Monitor
S Surgeon
A1 First assistant
N Nurse

Fig. 4.1 Position of operating personnel and trocars and cannulae for routine gynaecological laparoscopic surgery.

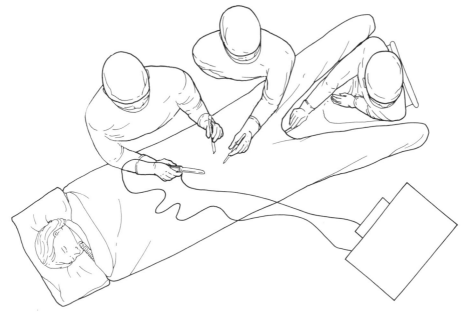

Fig. 4.2 Position of surgeon and assistant during standard laparoscopic surgery.

times it may be necessary to look through another portal and so the surgeon must be able to adapt to working from different aspects of the pelvis. Initially this may prove to be quite difficult. The position of the patient may cause confusion at first — she will usually be in a fairly steep Trendelenburg position and may also be tilted laterally. This will alter the surgeon's perspective.

It is important to identify the pelvic organs accurately and to plan the insertion of the secondary trocars and cannulae to avoid injury to bowel, bladder or ureter.

When using electric or laser energy or when using scissors or forceps it is essential to take any steps necessary to avoid possible injury.

Site of secondary portals

At least two secondary portals are necessary through which ancillary instruments may be introduced. On occasion, it may be necessary to establish a fourth or even a fifth portal.

1 Most laparoscopic surgery can be performed through the 'safety triangle' which has its apex at the umbilicus and its base at the pubic symphysis. Its lateral walls are the line of the obliterated umbilical artery on either side (Fig. 4.3). Incisions within this triangle will usually avoid the deep inferior epigastric arteries, which are frequently at risk of damage when trocars and cannulae are being inserted through the abdominal wall.

2 The incisions should be far enough apart so that the instruments do not get in each other's way and provide a reasonable divergent

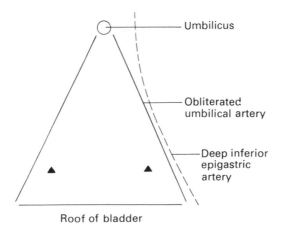

Fig. 4.3 The safety triangle bounded by the obliterated umbilical arteries and the pubic symphysis.

angle. They should be low enough to be cosmetic but high enough to allow the instruments to reach behind the uterus into the pouch of Douglas. The upper line of the pubic hair about 4 cm above the symphysis is usually a satisfactory site but may be too low if there is extensive deep endometriosis.

3 A more lateral incision is sometimes necessary. Making the safety triangle incisions always entails passing the trocar and cannula through the rectus abdominis muscle, which is satisfactory for most purposes and it is rare to produce an incisional hernia. However, if repeated insertion of cannulae is necessary, a more lateral incision is preferable as it is easier to find the same pathway through the external oblique muscle. In this case McBurney's point or its equivalent on the left side is a useful insertion site.

4 The presence of multiple adhesions may dictate the choice of an alternative site which will be governed by the position of the adhesions and the organ to be treated.

5 The portals should be far enough from the target tissues to allow easy approach with scissors or forceps. If an adhesion is too close to the portal of entry it may be impossible to divide it.

Haemostasis

During any surgical procedure it is essential to be able to prevent or control bleeding. In laparoscopic surgery there is often less bleeding than in conventional surgery because:

1 The intra-abdominal pressure, which is usually 15 mmHg, is higher than the venous pressure and therefore bleeding from small vessels tends to stop very quickly.

2 Warm lavage solution has a haemostatic effect.

3 The view of the target tissue is better than during laparotomy because of the proximity of the laparoscope lens and the magnification produced by the telescope and the video screen. Thus vessels can be easily seen and coagulated or ligated before transection. Small bleeding points may be identified by submerging them in irrigating fluid and putting the distal lens of the laparoscope below the surface. Their point of origin may be clearly identified using this method.

The easiest bleeding to control is that which has not yet occurred and the surgeon should aim to ensure this state of affairs by identifying vessels and occluding them prior to division. It is always preferable, where possible, to dissect vessels free from the surrounding tissue so that energy, ligatures or clips can be applied accurately. As with conventional surgery, the vessels should be occluded at two points and divided between them (Fig. 4.4). If bleeding does occur, the vessels should be identified and grasped with forceps. This will temporarily arrest the bleeding while a decision is made about the most appropriate method of ensuring permanent control.

It is always preferable to ensure that blood vessels are occluded before they are divided. Nevertheless, occasions will arise when bleeding occurs and must be stopped. Haemostasis may be achieved by coagulation using bipolar or monopolar current, thermal energy

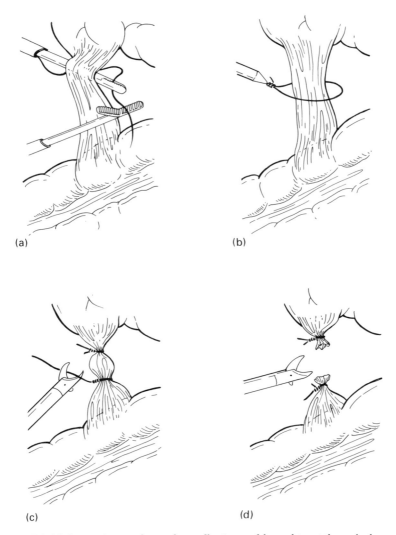

(a)

(b)

(c)

(d)

Fig. 4.4 (a) Suture is passed round an adhesion and brought out through the cannula to be tied extra-corporeally; (b) the knot is pushed down to tighten it; (c) two ligatures are applied and the sutures cut; (d) the adhesion is divided between the two ligatures.

or by ligation with sutures or clips. Injection of vasoconstrictive solutions may be valuable. Lasers are less effective.

Bipolar electrocoagulation. The current passes from one blade of the coagulating forceps to the other with no spread of electric current through adjacent tissues but with a certain amount of lateral transmission of heat. There is, therefore, no danger of distant burns but there is danger of thermal damage to nearby structures. The vessel to be coagulated should be identified and grasped between the blades. The surgeon ensures that the blades are not in contact with any other vital structures. The current is passed until the vessel blanches or the current ceases to flow, indicating dessication of the tissues. Larger vessels may need to be coagulated twice.

Monopolar electrocoagulation. The coagulating current is applied to the target tissue with an electrode or forceps and must then return to the dispersive plate along other tissue planes (Fig. 4.5). It is during this return that the electric current may cause a burn outside the operator's visual field, which may result in a bowel or ureteric fistula. Monopolar current should not be used to control bleeding from major vessels but it is useful for spot coagulation of small bleeding points.

Thermocoagulation. Thermocoagulation is effected by grasping the tissue with the blades of forceps or applying a point coagulator. Electric current heats the instrument to 120–140°C but does not then pass through the body. Thermocoagulation is safer in this

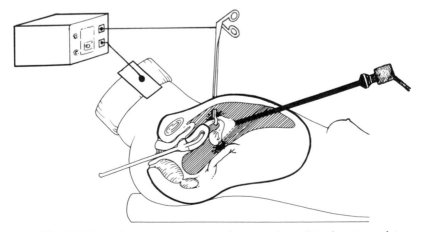

Fig. 4.5 Monopolar current may cause burns on its path to the return plate.

respect but is slower and may not coagulate as deeply as bipolar current and is less useful for dealing with large vessels.

Ligatures

Ligatures may be applied to a pedicle with a modified Roeder loop (endoloop) or the knot may be tied either inside or outside the body (intra- or extra-corporeal knotting).

The Roeder loop was originally described for use during paediatric tonsillectomy. It consists of a plastic applicator with a snap-off end and a loop of suture material with a pre-tied slip knot. The ligature

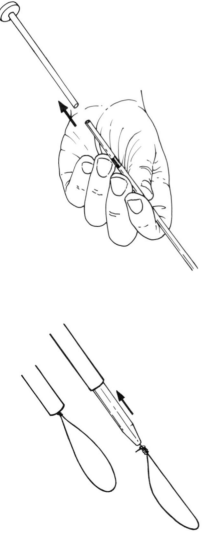

Fig. 4.6 Loading the Roeder loop into its applicator.

is inserted into the abdomen through an introducing channel which fits into a standard 5 mm cannula. The technique of application to a pedicle is as follows:

1 The loop and applicator are back loaded into the introducer by inserting its proximal end through the distal end of the applicator channel. The applicator is advanced until the loop is completely within the introducer (Fig. 4.6).

2 The introducer containing the endoloop is inserted into the abdomen through a 5 mm cannula. The plastic applicator is advanced until the loop is seen. The loop is placed over the pedicle.

3 A grasping forceps is inserted through a contra-lateral cannula. Its tip is positioned within the loop (Fig. 4.7).

4 The pedicle is grasped and drawn upwards through the loop.

5 The small end-piece of the applicator is snapped off. The end-piece is pulled back while, at the same time, the applicator is slid forwards, thus pushing the knot down on to the pedicle. The ligature is positioned on the pedicle by a combination of manipulating the grasper and tightening the endoloop.

6 The grasping forceps are removed and both hands are used to tighten the ligature and achieve complete haemostasis.

7 The grasping forceps are replaced by scissors and the ligature cut about 0.5 cm from the knot (Fig. 4.8).

8 If the pedicle is thick, one or two more ligatures should be applied.

Suturing techniques

Sutures may be inserted laparoscopically and the knots tied outside the abdomen (extra-corporeal knotting) or inside (intra-corporeal knotting).

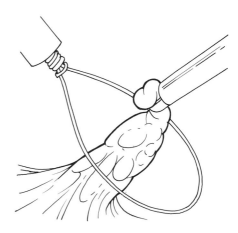

Fig. 4.7 Applying the Roeder loop around a bleeding pedicle.

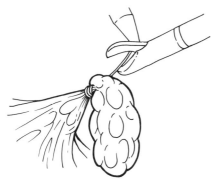

Fig. 4.8 Cutting the ligature after it has been tightened.

In *extra-corporeal knotting*, the suture is passed through the tissue and then brought outside the abdomen through the cannula to tie the knot. The ligature is available pre-packed with a sterile plastic applicator, suture and straight needle. The suture is placed as follows:

1 The needle and suture are held in the needle holder close to the attachment of the needle to the suture (swage point) and loaded into the introducer. The needle falls back on itself so that the sharp point is introduced last (Fig. 4.9).

2 The introducer is inserted into the abdomen through a 5 mm cannula until the needle is seen.

3 Grasping forceps are introduced through a contralateral channel. The needle is taken by the grasping forceps (Fig. 4.10a).

4 The needle holder now grasps the needle at the desired point and the needle angle is altered with the grasper until it is perpendicular to the axis of the holder. The grasper is disengaged (Fig. 4.10b).

5 The needle is passed through the tissue. The tip is taken by the grasping forceps and the needle pulled through the tissue. The

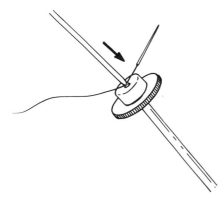

Fig. 4.9 Introducing a straight needle by holding it close to the swage point.

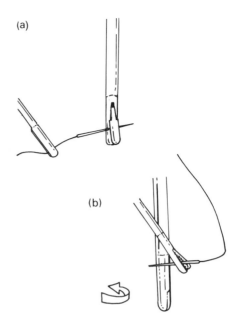

Fig. 4.10 (a) Catching the needle with the grasping forceps; (b) altering the angle of the needle.

forceps may be used to depress the tissue if there is difficulty locating the tip (Fig. 4.11).

6 The needle is passed back to the needle holder, taking care to hold the sharp tip within the jaws of the holder. More suture length is pulled into the abdomen with the grasper. The suture is pulled through the tissue, taking care not to pull on the suture line.

7 The needle is withdrawn from the abdomen by holding it close to the swage point. Both ends of the suture are now outside the abdomen.

8 An assistant should cover the end of the cannula with a finger to prevent loss of pneumoperitoneum. The knot may now be tied.

9 A single throw knot is made and the knot held between thumb and third finger (Fig. 4.12).

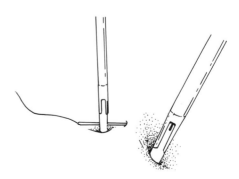

Fig. 4.11 Inserting a straight needle whilst depressing the tissues with the grasping forceps.

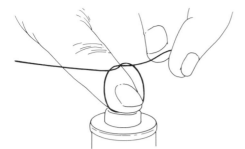

Fig. 4.12 Extra-corporeal knotting: making a single throw knot with the two suture ends.

10 The free end is brought round both strands of the suture three times (Fig. 4.13).

11 The free end is brought between the strands and then inserted through the loop which was formed by the first single throw knot. The knot is completed by pulling up on the free end (Fig. 4.14). The free end is cut about 0.5 cm from the knot.

12 The applicator is then inserted into the abdomen through the introducing cannula, its short plastic end snapped off and the knot tightened in the same fashion as the Roeder loop. The ligature is cut 0.5 cm from the knot.

Intra-corporeal knotting is a standard technique which should be learnt by all surgeons. Initially, it is technically difficult. Its use in some circumstances is debatable. A straight needle may be introduced into the abdomen through a 5 mm cannula or passed through the abdominal wall and grasped with a needle holder. The disadvantage of this is that a straight needle has limited use when suturing tissues such as the ovary or myometrium. A ski needle overcomes

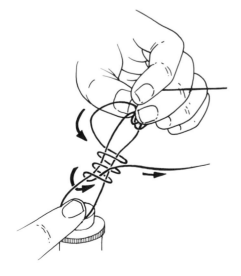

Fig. 4.13 Extra-corporeal knotting: the completed suture.

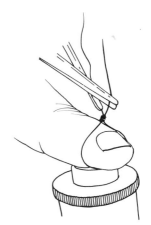

Fig. 4.14 Extra-corporeal knotting: the short end is cut prior to pushing the knot into the abdomen.

some of these disadvantages but it is possible to introduce a curved needle using only a standard 5 mm cannula.

The cannula is best sited laterally through the external oblique muscle which makes it easier to re-introduce it without the trocar. The technique is as follows:

1 The cannula is removed from the abdominal incision (Fig. 4.15a).

2 The needle holder is passed through the cannula and used to grasp the suture about 15 cm from the needle (Fig. 4.15b).

3 The cannula with the needle holder, but without its trocar, is re-introduced through the incision, carrying with it the suture which is on the outside of the cannula.

4 The cannula and needle holder are withdrawn. Grasping forceps are introduced through a contralateral portal and are used to grasp the suture and exert traction. The needle is pulled through the abdominal incision and into the peritoneal cavity (Fig. 4.15c).

5 The cannula and needle holder are re-introduced.

The suture should now be cut to the desired length. It is not possible to work with standard length sutures because of the limited space available within the abdomen.

The technique of suturing is as follows:

1 The needle is grasped with the needle holder at the desired position and held at right angles to the axis of the holder (Fig. 4.16).

2 The needle is passed through the tissue and held by the grasping forceps. A straight needle may be held in the grasping forceps whilst tying the knot. A curved needle may be 'parked' temporarily in the anterior abdominal wall peritoneum.

3 The suture is pulled through the tissue until about 5 cm remains.

4 The needle is held in the needle holder with its point facing in the direction of the short end of the suture (Fig. 4.17a). A short length of

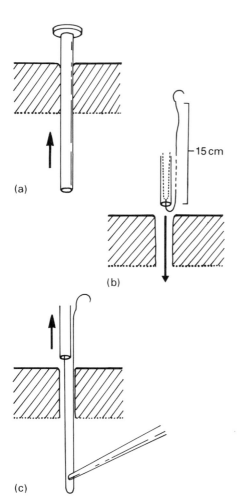

(a)

(b)

15 cm

(c)

Fig. 4.15 Introducing a curved needle using a 5 mm cannula: (a) the suture is grasped by the needle holder; (b) the cannula with needle holder is inserted into the abdomen; (c) the cannula is withdrawn and the needle pulled through the incision with grasping forceps.

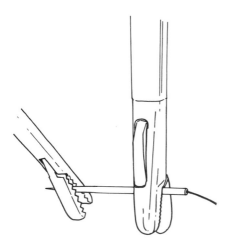

Fig. 4.16 Intra-corporeal knotting: the needle is held 5 mm from the swage point.

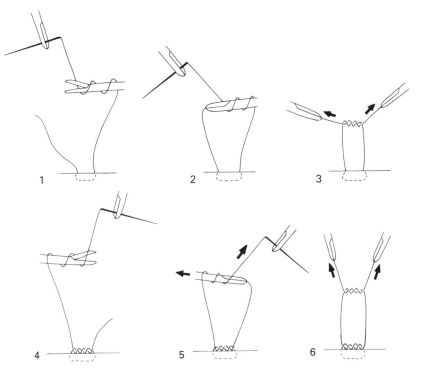

Fig. 4.17 Intra-corporeal knotting.

the needle should protrude from the holder to make knot tying easier. With the grasper between the suture and the surgeon, a double loop is made round the needle holder and the knot is pulled tight (Fig. 4.17, 1–3).

5 The needle is now held in the grasper with its point in the same direction as the short end of the suture (Fig. 4.17, 4–6). A double loop is made around the needle holder with the holder between the suture and the surgeon. The knot is pulled tight to complete the surgical knot. This produces a flat knot.

6 Both ends of the suture are held with the grasper 4 cm from the knot. The needle holder is removed and replaced with scissors. The suture is cut 0.5 cm from the knot.

7 The needle is removed either through the cannula or, in the case of a curved needle, by removing the cannula and pulling it through the incision.

Using these techniques, suture material as fine as 6/0 may be used for fine ovarian or tubal surgery and 1–3/0 for other applications. Catgut should never be used. Either fine nylon or PDS sutures are less likely to cause tissue reaction. If possible the knot should be tied so that it is buried beneath the surface of the tissue so the least possible suture material is exposed to the abdominal cavity.

Clips and staples

A variety of haemostatic clips are available which may be applied to vessels by disposable or re-usable applicators. While they are used less frequently, they can be invaluable to occlude vessels in situations where the use of high frequency current, thermocoagulation or the placement of sutures may be difficult or impossible.

Staples have enabled more advanced laparoscopic surgery to be performed more easily. Most of the staples available are introduced by disposable applicators which are, of necessity, expensive. The device is applied over the tissue to be divided and when it is closed, three lines of staples are automatically inserted on each side of a cutting knife. Thus, when the structure is divided haemostasis has already been secured by a triple row of staples. The disadvantage of the currently available instruments is that the staples do not reach to the tip of the applicator. There may, therefore, be bleeding beyond its tip. Staples are not suitable to occlude a vessel which is already bleeding.

Vasoconstriction

Haemostasis may be produced by the injection of the vasoconstricting agents vasopressin or adrenaline. This is of value in situations where there is increased vascularity such as in the conservative treatment of tubal pregnancy, the treatment of ovarian endometriosis and in myomectomy. In an ectopic pregnancy the injection should be at the point of entry of the vascular supply. In myomectomy the entire operation site should be infiltrated.

Vasopressin (POR 8, Sandoz) is injected in a concentration of 5 IU in 100 ml of normal saline. Usually two or three injections of 10 ml of solution is sufficient to produce satisfactory haemostasis. The site of action of POR 8 is on the terminal arterioles supplying the capillary network. Larger vessels are not affected and will bleed when divided. It is therefore essential when using vasoconstricting drugs to coagulate any visible bleeding vessel even when the bleeding is slight and would be controlled by warm lavage in other circumstances. Failure to control bleeding may lead to significant reactionary haemorrhage when the action of the drug wears off, which is usually within 30 minutes.

Alternatively, adrenaline in a concentration of 1 : 200 000 may be used but this has the disadvantage of occasionally producing cardiac arrhythmia and also is more likely to be followed by a reactionary hyperaemia so that bleeding may occur some time after surgery has been completed.

Laser

Carbon dioxide laser is the most commonly used for laparoscopic surgery, and in many respects the most useful. It has excellent precise cutting properties but will only control minor oozing. When using CO_2 laser it is imperative, therefore, to have available either thermocoagulation or bipolar electrocoagulation capability. The Nd : YAG laser, on the other hand, is haemostatic but has the disadvantage that it penetrates deeply and may damage tissues underlying the target organ.

Prevention of adhesions

The principles of prevention of adhesions in laparoscopic surgery are similar to those which apply in conventional surgery:
1 Gentle tissue handling.
2 Keep tissues moist. This is probably easier in laparoscopic surgery because the operation is performed in a closed environment with less chance of tissue drying.
3 Control of haemostasis.
4 Accurate approximation of tissues. This is more difficult because of the limitations on accurate suturing.
5 The appropriate choice of suture material and the correct placement of knots.
6 Use of adjuvants which may help to prevent adhesion formation, such as fibrin glue and heparinized saline solution.

Fibrin glue. A commercially available solution, 'Tisseel kit' (Fig. 4.18), may be used to cover oozing areas of tissue and aid promotion of haemostasis. 'Tisseel' may also be used instead of sutures to close tissues such as the ovary following ovariotomy or to re-peritonize the pelvis after treatment of endometriosis or hysterectomy. The vials of Aprotinin and Tisseel are heated for 10 minutes in a water bath at 37°C, mixed, agitated and heated again for 10–15 minutes. The thrombin and calcium chloride are mixed separately at 37°C. The solutions are applied to the tissues using a needle and special double syringe system. The tissues are held together with forceps for 3–5 minutes to ensure that the sealant adheres firmly to the surrounding

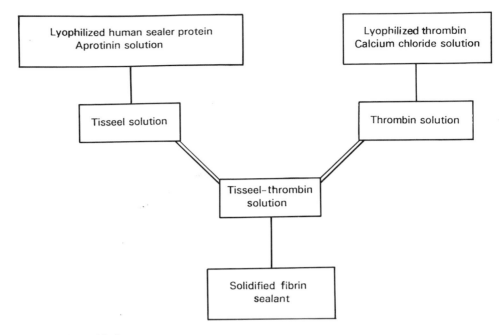

Fig. 4.18 'Tisseel kit'.

tissue. The sealant reaches 70% of its ultimate strength within 10 minutes and its full strength in about 2 hours.

Principles of adhesiolysis

Adhesiolysis may be performed with scissors, a monopolar micro-needle or laser. In all cases it is essential that the adhesion be divided as close as possible to its attachment and not in the middle of the adhesion.

In general, adhesiolysis should commence at the abdominal wall and proceed caudally towards the pouch of Douglas. However, if there are extensive abdominal adhesions it may only be possible to divide them from below upwards and in this case it may be helpful to use a 5 mm laparoscope through one of the lower incisions to improve access.

Careful study of the adhesions will usually reveal an avascular area to divide, but if there are any vessels they should be coagulated before division. The scissors, micro-needle or laser should always approach the adhesion at right angles. The most appropriate portal should be chosen to achieve this objective. Traction should be placed on the adhesions by atraumatic forceps to position the adhesion correctly. Scissor dissection may be close to the organ but electric energy or laser should be applied 1–2 mm away from the organ to

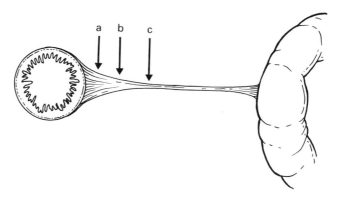

Fig. 4.19 Site of division of adhesion close to the fallopian tube: (a) scissors; (b) laser; (c) electrosurgery.

prevent damage by lateral spread of heat (Fig. 4.19). For the same reason, only blunt or scissor dissection should be used when two organs, such as loops of bowel, are adherent to each other with no appreciable space between them.

Hydrodissection

Lavage with a warm solution of heparinized Ringer lactate solution is an essential part of laparoscopic surgery. Hydrostatic pressure may also be used to dissect tissues. The fluid may be injected and aspirated through a simple cannula which is equipped with a two-way tap. More sophisticated systems (Triton, Aquadissector) are attached to automated pumps allowing irrigation and suction and contain a channel through which a retractable monopolar needle may be inserted. The tip of the cannula is placed behind the adhesion, either through a natural tissue plane or through a small incision close to its attachment. When the fluid is turned on it will find the path of least resistance and effectively and atraumatically create a line of dissection without risk of perforating the adjacent organs. The adhesion may now be divided by blunt dissection using the tip of the cannula, scissors, micro-needle or laser.

Hydrodissection may also be used to provide a fluid backstop for carbon dioxide laser. In this case, a small incision is made in the peritoneum and the tip of the flushing cannula inserted. Irrigation fluid will flow deep to the peritoneum, lifting it from underlying structures. The fluid will now prevent damage by laser to these structures.

Peritoneal lavage is used to remove blood, fibrin and debris and to keep the tissues moist. This helps to prevent adhesion formation. The tissues must be kept moist at all times using copious amounts of physiological solutions maintained at a temperature of 37–40°C. Fluid, smoke, blood and debris must be evacuated during surgery. It may be necessary to reverse the Trendelenburg position to remove fluid from the upper abdomen.

Removal of tissues from the abdomen

It is essential to remove all excised tissues at the completion of the operation. Small pieces of tissue may be removed along a 5 mm cannula. Frequently, these cannulae are too small. Several techniques may be used to remove larger pieces:

1 A cystic structure may be aspirated and then removed.
2 The tissue may be cut into smaller pieces with scissors or morcellated with a tissue punch.
3 The tissue may be cut longitudinally to reduce its diameter and then removed through an 11 mm cannula.
4 The tissue may be grasped with forceps and then guided into the primary cannula under visual control and removed.
5 An abdominal suprapubic incision may be enlarged to accommodate the tissue.
6 The umbilical incision may be enlarged and the tissue removed through it under visual control by a laparoscope inserted through one of the lower incisions.
7 A cruciate incision may be made in the posterior vaginal fornix and the tissue removed vaginally.

Removal of instruments

Finally, all instruments and cannulae must be removed from the abdomen. It is important that this is always done under direct vision or an organ may be accidentally included in the jaws of forceps and damaged by pulling it into the cannula or incision.

Suture of incisions

All the wounds must be sutured or closed with clips at the completion of the operation. Incisions larger than 5 mm should be closed in two layers to prevent hernia formation.

Conclusion

Strict adherence to these principles should result in safe, satisfying and effective surgery. Ignoring these principles may lead the surgeon into a morass of complications.

5: Simple Laparoscopic Surgery

Tubal interruption
  Thermal destruction
  Mechanical obstruction
Simple adhesiolysis
Aspiration of ovarian cyst

Coagulation of endometriosis and
  peritoneal biopsy
Polycystic ovarian disease
Uterine ventrosuspension
Salpingectomy

The laparoscopic surgeon in training should start by performing simple procedures which involve insertion of one or more ancillary instruments, so experience can be gained in three dimensional working from a video screen without risk of damaging any vital organs. The simplest and easiest operation is to effect sterilization by tubal interruption.

Tubal interruption

Tubal interruption may be effected by:
1 Thermal destruction
  (a) Monopolar electrocoagulation
  (b) Bipolar electrocoagulation
  (c) Thermocoagulation
  (d) Laser
2 Mechanical obstruction
  (a) Tubal clips
  (b) Fallope ring
3 Salpingectomy
  (a) Ligation
  (b) Bipolar coagulation and excision

Thermal destruction

Monopolar electrocoagulation. The classical method of monopolarelectrocoagulation with or without division of the tube has now fallen into disrepute and should not be performed. A high frequency current was used to dessicate the tubal isthmus (Fig. 5.1). However, on a number of occasions the current caused damage to other organs on its return path to the dispersive plate. This resulted in burns to the bowel with resulting faecal fistulae or damage to the ureter or bladder. Occasionally, there were burns to the patient's skin when

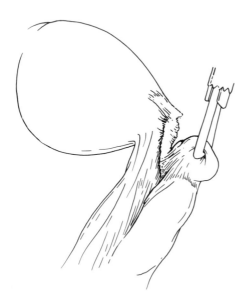

Fig. 5.1 Monopolar electrocoagulation and division of the fallopian tube.

the instruments were not properly insulated and it was even possible for the surgeon to suffer burns to the face or hands if the patient was not earthed properly.

Bipolar electrocoagulation avoids many of the hazards of the monopolar operation although there is still a risk of damaging adjacent structures by direct transmission of heat. In this operation, the bipolar forceps are introduced through a second portal of entry and used to grasp the tubal isthmus. The blades of the forceps are placed in such a fashion that the full diameter of the tube is included and the tips extend to the mesosalpinx (Fig. 5.2). The tube is drawn upwards to isolate it and ensure that no other organ is in contact

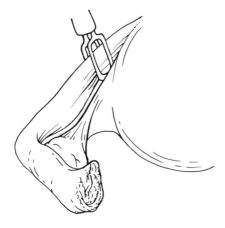

Fig. 5.2 Bipolar electrocoagulation: the isthmus of the tube is grasped and drawn upwards.

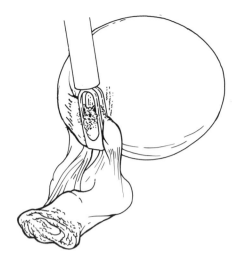

Fig. 5.3 Bipolar electrocoagulation: a segment of the tube is coagulated.

with or near to the fallopian tube. The current is applied and maintained until the tube is seen to bubble and collapse. Ideally, a flow meter should be used to indicate when the current stops flowing and dessication is complete. Bipolar coagulation may be applied in one or two more areas until about 2 cm of the tubal isthmus has been destroyed (Fig. 5.3).

The forceps blades are opened and gently disengaged under visual control. Occasionally, the tube adheres to the forceps. As efforts to dislodge the forceps may cause tearing and bleeding, the tube and mesosalpinx should be thoroughly inspected once the forceps have been freed. If bleeding is noted, the vessel should be grasped and coagulated. Constantly keeping the forceps in view, they are moved to the other side of the pelvis and the contra-lateral tube is occluded.

Some surgeons transect the coagulated tube with scissors but, while this ensures that the two ends of the coagulated tube fall apart, it may cause a tubal fistula and lead to failure of the sterilization (Fig. 5.4). The length of tube which has been destroyed makes tubal reconstruction less likely to succeed.

Thermocoagulation is probably safer than either of the above procedures because no electric current passes into the body and the temperature produced is much lower than with electrocoagulation. For this reason it is possible that the full thickness of the tube may not be destroyed and so the failure rate is likely to be higher. The details of this technique are identical to those described for bipolar electrocoagulation, but division of the tube with scissors is usually recommended when thermocoagulation is used.

Once the tubes have been satisfactorily coagulated, the forceps are

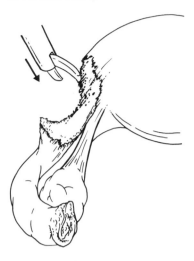

Fig. 5.4 Bipolar electrocoagulation: the coagulated area is divided with scissors.

removed and a pair of scissors inserted. The blades are opened at the mid-point of the coagulated area and closed to divide the tube, while avoiding the underlying mesosalpinx and the tubal vessels. If a mesosalpingeal vessel does bleed, the scissors are removed, replaced with coagulating forceps and haemostasis is secured before proceeding to divide the contra-lateral tube.

Mechanical obstruction

Tubal clips. A variety of mechanical tubal clips have been designed to occlude the tube without the risk of thermal damage to surrounding tissues.

The *Filshie clip* (Fig. 5.5a) is made of titanium with a silastic lining. Closure is effected by the upper jaw being seated in a notch in the distal end of the lower jaw. The tube is compressed by expansion of the silastic.

The *Hulka–Clemens clip* (Fig. 5.5b) is made of Lexon, a transparent plastic, with a stainless steel hinge and a gold-plated stainless steel spring. The force of closure of the clip on the tube depends on the tensile strength of the spring.

Each clip is applied with a specially designed applicator. Both applicators carry the clip in a distal groove. The Filshie clip is closed by a jaw-like mechanism. The Hulka clip is closed by a piston closing the clip and pushing the spring forwards. In both, the control is effected proximally. Although there are minor variations in technique depending on which type of clip is used, the basic principles are the same.

The clip is placed across the isthmus of the tube and partially

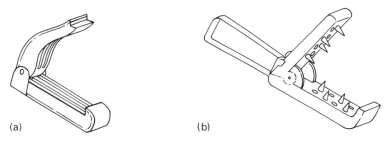

Fig. 5.5 (a) The Filshie clip; (b) the Hulka–Clemens clip.

closed (Fig. 5.6). The applicator is slightly withdrawn and rotated so the surgeon can be assured that the clip has been applied vertically to the full diameter of the tube. Once satisfied that the application is accurate, the clip is locked and the applicator withdrawn from the tube. The tip of the applicator is used as a blunt probe with which the tube is manipulated so that correct application can be confirmed. The applicator is removed, a second clip is loaded and the procedure repeated on the other side.

Complications of this operation are uncommon. The tube may be torn and bleed at the site of application if manipulation is not gentle or if removal of the clip is attempted. In this case, application of a second clip may control the bleeding or it may be controlled by

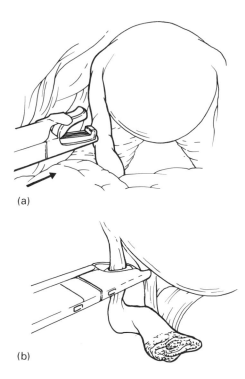

Fig. 5.6 (a) The Filshie clip approaches the isthmus of the left fallopian tube; (b) the applicator is rotated to ensure that the clip is correctly applied.

electrocoagulation. The Hulka clip is easily removed by a sharp pull, but the Filshie clip locks on to the tube and should not be removed because of the risk of tearing and bleeding. This may usually be avoided by careful inspection of the clip both during and after application. Misapplication of the clip may lead to failure of the sterilization. The failure rate of this operation is small (approximately 3 : 1000) but could be improved by applying two clips close together on the isthmus. If the clips are far apart it is possible for a small hydrosalpinx to develop which could be a cause of post-operative pain and would also necessitate excision of a greater length of tube if subsequent reversal of sterilization were requested.

Fallope ring. The fallope ring was also devised to overcome the problems of electro-coagulation. The ring is made from silastic rubber impregnated with barium sulphate to make it radio-opaque. It has an external diameter of 3.1 mm and an internal diameter of 1.1 mm. It is applied with a special applicator, either through the channel of an operating laparoscope or through a secondary portal. The applicator has an outer sheath with a guard to hold one or two rings close to its tip. Within the sheath there is a retractile forceps with which to grasp the tube.

The ring is loaded on to the applicator using a cone-shaped attachment. The applicator is introduced into the abdomen and the forceps grasps the fallopian tube in the mid-isthmic segment (Fig. 5.7). A loop of tube is drawn up into the applicator by a combination of gentle traction and advancing the applicator over the loop (Fig. 5.8). When the loop is securely within the channel, the

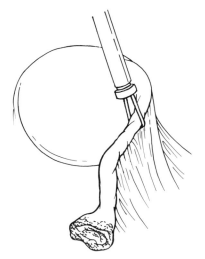

Fig. 5.7 Fallope ring: the applicator is applied to the mid-isthmic segment.

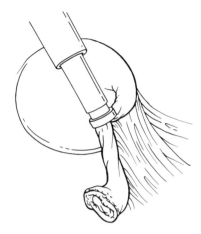

Fig. 5.8 Fallope ring: the applicator is advanced over the loop of the tube.

fallope ring is pushed off the end of the applicator and over the loop of tube (Fig. 5.9).

There is some risk of transecting the tube as it is drawn into the applicator, with consequent bleeding. If the tube is thick or fibrosed it may be impossible to apply the fallope ring and an alternative method should be employed.

Salpingectomy

Salpingectomy either by ligation or coagulation and excision is a more complex operation, it is discussed later in this chapter.

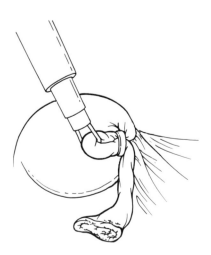

Fig. 5.9 Fallope ring: the Fallope ring is pushed off the end of the applicator and over the loop of the tube.

Simple adhesiolysis

The amount and density of adhesions varies from the mild to the very severe. Laparoscopic removal of very dense adhesive disease can be one of the most difficult and complex of all laparoscopic operations. Laparoscopic excision of fine avascular adhesions is relatively simple. The former will be described in the chapter on complex operative procedures; the latter provides the opportunity for the trainee to develop skills in advance of those required to perform sterilization. Removal of less dense adhesions between the tube and ovary (salpingo-ovariolysis) is an example of a relatively simple operation. If the complaint is of infertility, the results can be gratifying.

The laparoscope is inserted and an initial assessment of the adhesions made. If they are deemed resectable, two secondary portals should be introduced in the safety triangle on either side of the midline. Initially, grasping forceps are inserted through one of the secondary portals and the structures manipulated so that the extent of the adhesive disease can be thoroughly evaluated (Fig. 5.10). There is nearly always an avascular area at the attachment of the adhesion which should be identified. Scissors are inserted through the other secondary portal. The uterine manipulator and the grasping forceps are used to display the adhesion and put it on the stretch. The scissors are placed close to the attachment of the adhesion to the tube, and the lower blade is used to lift the adhesion so that it is free from any vital structures (Fig. 5.11). The adhesion is incised. If a blood vessel is noticed as the incision proceeds, the scissors are removed and replaced with the bipolar grasping forceps. The vessel is seized 1–2 mm from the tube and

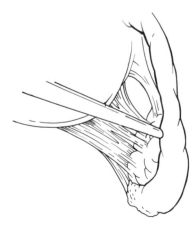

Fig. 5.10 Ovariolysis: the extent and attachments of the adhesion are thoroughly evaluated.

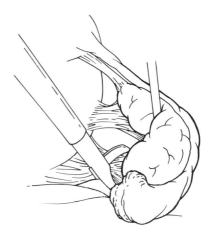

Fig. 5.11 Ovariolysis: the adhesion is displayed with the scissors before dividing it close to the ovary.

coagulated. The coagulating forceps are removed, the scissors replaced and the dissection proceeds. Once the adhesion has been completely freed from the tube, the grasping forceps are transferred to the free end and the other attachment is dissected free. The grasping forceps, still holding the now free fibrous tissue, are withdrawn, thus removing the adhesion from the abdominal cavity.

An alternative approach is to use a monopolar cutting point or laser. When these forms of energy are used, precautions must be taken to avoid damage to adjacent structures.

Division of adhesions close to the bowel or between loops of bowel should not be attempted too early in the learning process, as these can be the most difficult and potentially dangerous of operations.

Aspiration of ovarian cyst

If there is doubt about their nature, small ovarian cysts may be aspirated to obtain fluid for cytological examination. However, it would seem unnecessary to aspirate a physiological cyst and a pathological cyst will always recur after simple aspiration.

The ovarian ligament is held in forceps to steady the ovary which can then be punctured by a long spinal or Veress' needle. Alternatively, a 5 mm punction needle may be introduced through another secondary portal to aspirate the cyst (Fig. 5.12). The fluid should always be sent for cytological examination, but it should be remembered that this is not as accurate a means of detecting malignancy as histological examination of the cyst wall. The experienced surgeon will have learnt to open the cyst, assess it accurately to exclude malignancy and, if it is benign, remove it while conserving normal ovarian tissue.

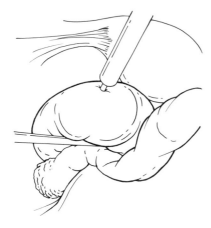

Fig. 5.12 Aspiration of an ovarian cyst using a 5 mm punction needle.

Coagulation of endometriosis and peritoneal biopsy

It is clear that destruction of small endometriotic implants exerts very little effect on the outcome for patients complaining of pain or infertility. Nevertheless, it is difficult to resist the temptation to do so. Despite our best assurances it is often impossible to persuade the majority of patients that leaving the disease untreated is in their best interests. It should be stated strongly that destruction of small endometriotic implants should only be performed if all of the visible lesion can be destroyed without putting any vital structure at risk.

Small implants of endometriosis may be coagulated with fine bipolar forceps or with the point coagulator of the endotherm. Care should be taken when working in proximity to the ureter, which should always be identified when the endometriosis is present on the pelvic side wall or broad ligament. It is necessary to coagulate not only the active plaques of endometriosis but also the abnormal vessels in the peritoneum surrounding the plaques, as these often contain active endometriosis.

A slightly more advanced procedure, but still a simple one, is to lift the peritoneum with forceps and then excise the endometriosis with a monopolar microneedle or scissors to obtain a biopsy specimen to confirm the diagnosis as well as remove the lesion.

Polycystic ovarian disease

In cases of polycystic ovarian disease, return of spontaneous ovulation often follows drilling of the multiple ovarian cysts with a monopolar needle or an argon or carbon dioxide laser. The ovary is held with forceps applied to the ovarian ligament which allows the ovary to be lifted and rotated to expose all its aspects. Each small cyst is drilled with the needle and a cutting/coagulating current used to destroy its lining. If the laser is used, the focused beam drills the wall and the defocused beam destroys the lining. The fluid which escapes from the cyst is washed away with copious peritoneal lavage.

The results of this simple operation are good in the short term in that ovulation and fertility are often restored for up to one year, but after that the ovulation defect usually recurs.

Uterine ventrosuspension

Uterine ventrosuspension was one of the first laparoscopic operations. It has largely fallen into disrepute. It is not indicated for simple uterine retroversion but may have merit in cases of deep dyspareunia and to prevent the uterus falling into the pouch of Douglas and possibly reforming adhesions following treatment of endometriosis.

Skin incisions about 2 cm long should be made bilaterally over the internal inguinal ring which is 2 cm above the inguinal ligament at the junction of its lateral and medial two thirds. The abdominal wall should be transilluminated at this point to avoid damaging vessels. An incision is made with a fine scalpel in the external oblique aponeurosis and toothed Kocher forceps thrust through the incision and the underlying peritoneum under visual control. The round ligament is grasped at its mid-point and a loop of ligament brought to the surface (Fig. 5.13). The procedure is repeated on the contra-lateral side.

The abdomen is deflated to restore the normal relationships of the uterus to the abdominal wall. Both ligaments are elevated by traction on the forceps and are transfixed with an absorbable suture. The suture is inserted into the ligament and firmly tied round it. The external oblique aponeurosis is then transfixed by the suture and the ligament fixed to it. Any redundant ligament may be excised with a scalpel. The incision in the abdomen is closed with subcutaneous

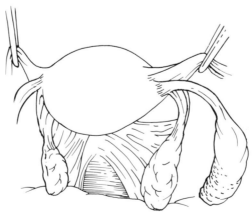

Fig. 5.13 Uterine ventrosuspension. The round ligament is grasped at its mid point and drawn through an incision at the internal inguinal ring.

sutures or clips. It is advisable to keep the patient in hospital overnight as there may be considerable pain following this operation.

Ventrosuspension may occasionally cause distortion of the fallopian tube so should not be performed in this manner in cases of infertility. If the patient is infertile, the procedure may be modified to prevent distortion. In this case the ligament should be brought to the surface and transfixed with a suture which is tied to allow the apex of the loop to remain within the peritoneal cavity. This produces less distortion but may not be so effective in anteverting the uterus.

Salpingectomy

The surgeon who has gained proficiency in these techniques should now be ready to proceed to salpingectomy using the principles already mastered in operating off the video screen and using instruments introduced through secondary cannulae. Salpingectomy may be indicated to treat an ectopic pregnancy or for tubal sterilization. In either case the fallopian tube may be removed by ligation or by electrocoagulation. In the case of ectopic pregnancy, salpingectomy must be preceeded by pelvic lavage to remove blood and clots and gain access to the tube.

Ectopic pregnancy

The diagnosis of early ectopic pregnancy may be suspected when the patient has an altered menstrual pattern and is confirmed by serum βHCG estimation and transvaginal ultrasound scan. Although some 80% of tubal pregnancies may be diagnosed prior to rupture and treated conservatively as described in Chapter 6, many are diagnosed only after irreversible tubal damage has occurred. Salpingectomy is then the only possible treatment. This may be performed laparoscopically provided the patient is haemodynamically stable, the blood loss is less than two litres and the pregnancy is in the tubal isthmus or ampulla. A shocked patient should always be resuscitated prior to surgery. Laparoscopy carries a greater risk than laparotomy in a shocked patient because the elevation of the diaphragm by the pneumoperitoneum may cause further cardiac embarrassment. Excessive blood loss may lead to shock and it may also be very difficult to evacuate a large volume of blood with clots to obtain a clear view of the tubes. The site of the ectopic is important. An intramusral or cornual pregnancy is unsuitable for laparoscopic surgery because of the risk of torrential bleeding from the uterine atery and the need to excise a wedge of uterus and resuture it. This is tecnically difficult.

Laparoscopy is performed and the diagnosis confirmed. Two

secondary trocars and cannulae are inserted within the safety triangle and the pelvic organs examined using atraumatic grasping forceps to retract bowel and expose the tube. A 5 mm flushing tube is introduced through the contralateral cannula and blood aspirated, clots broken down and thorough pelvic lavage with warm Ringer lactate solution performed. If there is active bleeding the tube should be grasped with the forceps to control it temporarily. Salpingectomy may then be performed.

Loop ligation may be performed using a modified Roeder loop as described in Chapter 4. The loop is backloaded into its introducing cannula and inserted into the abdomen through a 5 mm cannula on the side of the ectopic pregnancy. The loop is placed over the tubal ampulla. The atraumatic forceps introduced through the contralateral 5 mm cannula then grasp the fimbrial end of the tube through the loop. The tube is then drawn upwards through the loop. The endoloop is manipulated until it is positioned around the fallopian tube proximal to the pregnancy. This may be difficult and can be assisted by introducing a second forceps or a long Veress'needle. The plastic end-piece is snapped off and the endoloop tightened by a combination of traction on the end piece and sliding the applicator forwards. When the knot is tight the forceps should be removed and replaced by scissors with which the ligature is divided about 0.5 cm from the knot. Two further endoloops should be applied to ensure haemostasis. These are inserted in the same fashion and the knot sited proximal to the first loop.

When the tube has been ligated, salpingectomy can be performed. The ligated tube is held with the atraumatic forceps introduced through the contralateral cannula and 5 mm scissors are introduced through the ipsilateral cannula. The tubal isthmus is carefully divided distal to the ligatures and the cut tube inspected to ensure that there is no bleeding. Section of the pedicle may now be completed with scisssors and the excised tube with its ectopic pregnancy 'parked' in the pouch of Douglas pending later removal.

Peritoneal lavage with warm Ringer lactate solution is now repeated until the pelvis is clean and the surgeon is satisfied that haemostasis is complete.

Electrocoagulation of the tube and mesosalpinx may be performed to obtain haemostasis prior to excision. Following laparoscopy and pelvic lavage, the tube is grasped just proximal to the ectopic pregnancy with bipolar forceps introduced through the contralateral 5 mm cannula. Bipolar forceps are inserted through the ipsilateral cannula. They are used to coagulate the tubal isthmus until it blanches. The bipolar forceps are removed and replaced by scissors with which the isthmus is divided. The initial incision should be made with the point of the scissors so that the tube can be inspected before complete division and the surgeon may be sure that dessication of the tube is complete. If the tube looks pink or bleeds, the coagulation should be repeated prior to complete division of the tube. The scissors are then removed, the bipolar forceps replaced and coagulation and division proceeds sequentially along the mesosalpinx towards the fimbria ovaricae until the tube has been completely removed from its attachment. The excised tube may then be stored in the pouch of Douglas pending removal from the abdomen. Peritoneal lavage should then be carried out with copious warm Ringer lactate solution.

Removal of the tube must now be performed. The tube is usually too large to be removed through a 5 mm cannula. One of the 5 mm cannulae may be removed and replaced with a 11 mm cannula and the ectopic pregnancy drawn through it. Frequently the pregnancy is too large to pass through the large cannula. In this case the tube should be held with the 11 mm grasping forceps and cut longitudinally with 5 mm scissors so that its diameter is halved. The majority of ectopic pregnancies may then be removed through the 11 mm cannula but occasionally it is necessary to carry out further morcellation to reduce its bulk and allow removal. It should never be necessary to enlarge the abdominal incision or to deliver it through the posterior vaginal fornix.

Finally peritoneal lavage is repeated to ensure haemostasis and leave the pelvis free of blood. The instruments should be removed from the abdomen under direct vision and the incisions sutured in one or two layers depending on the size of the incision.

Sterilization

The technique of sterilization by salpingectomy is similar. Laparoscopy is performed in the same way, two secondary trocars and cannulae are inserted through the safety triangle and salpingectomy performed either using endoloops or by coagulationa and division of the tube and mesosalpinx. Sterilization is easier than salpingectomy for ectopic pregnancy because there is no bleeding and the tube is smaller and easier to manipulate. Removal from the abdomen is also easier and can usually be accomplished through a 5 mm cannula. The small skin incisions should be sutured. The patient may usually be discharged from hospital on the same day.

6: Complex Laparoscopic Surgery

Introduction

Surgeons in training should increase their experience, initially under supervision, step by step until they have mastered all the standard procedures. These include multi-portal operating from a video screen, the use of mechanical, electro- and, when available, laser surgery. When they are confident that they are able to perform the procedures described in Chapter 5, they should be ready to proceed to more complex and difficult operations.

Neosalpingostomy

The classical treatment of distal tubal obstruction has been the use of microsurgical techniques which allow accurate assessment of the status of the fimbriae and provide the optimum conditions to operate efficiently with minimal tissue trauma. Nevertheless, good results are obtained in the distal tube without magnification and, more recently, equally good results have been obtained with laparoscopic surgery. There is no reported difference in outcome between laser and electro-mechanical surgery.

Prior detailed assessment of the status of the tube should have been made by hysterosalpingography (HSG) and, if previous diagnostic laparoscopy has been performed, by salpingoscopy and possibly by radionuclide hysterosalpingography (RNHSG). The results of surgery are largely dependent on the condition of the tubal mucosa and wall, the morphology and function of which can be assessed accurately by these means. However, while surgery gives the best results in tubal obstruction where the mucosa has been graded 1 or 2, occasional pregnancies have been obtained by surgery on tubes graded 3 and even 4. There is therefore some debate about whether or not to offer surgery in moderately damaged tubes. There is no place for surgery in cases of grade 5 tubal damage.

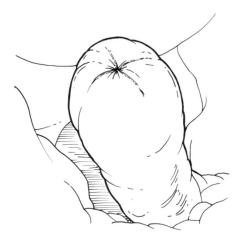

Fig. 6.1 Distal tubal
obstruction: the star shaped
scar is identified.

In many centres, distal tubal blockage is treated by laparotomy
and microsurgery. If laparoscopic distal tubal surgery becomes the
normal surgical approach for the unit, any case of simple diagnostic
laparoscopy for infertility could become a complex laparoscopic
procedure which may take 1–2 hours to perform. This may upset
operating room schedules, so staff and colleagues must be prepared
to be flexible in their arrangements.

Diagnostic laparoscopy is first performed and, as always, includes
a detailed examination of the abdominal cavity and pelvis. When
there is distal tubal blockage there are often associated peritubal
adhesions. These must be divided to gain access to the tubes and to
align them with the laparoscope and other instruments. When distal
blockage is diagnosed it is helpful to perform hydropertubation with
normal saline to distend the tube, and thus confirm proximal tubal

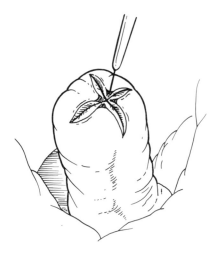

Fig. 6.2 Distal tubal obstruction:
3–4 radial incisions are made
through the avascular area of
obstructed distal end.

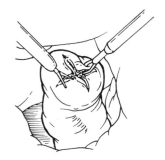

Fig. 6.3 Distal tubal obstruction: the incisions are extended using fine scissors.

patency, but not to discolour the mucosa with methylene blue, which hinders subsequent assessment of its condition. The star-shaped scar of the occluded distal end of the tube is now easily identified and can be incised (Fig. 6.1). The preliminary incisions should be made with a monopolar microneedle with the power setting as low as possible, usually about 5–10 watts. The incision should not be made through the full thickness of the tube, because this will cause the hydrosalpinx to collapse and make the operation more difficult to perform. As in microsurgery, there should be about three or four radial incisions through the avascular areas of the obstructed distal end (Fig. 6.2) following which the tube should be opened in the centre of the scar and the mucosa inspected using a salpingoscope (Chapter 3).

The incision may now be extended using fine scissors to open up the terminal end of the tube and expose the fimbriae (Fig. 6.3). The formation of the new opening may be completed using atraumatic forceps to tease it open in the same way as glass rods may be used in conventional surgery (Fig. 6.4). When the opening is deemed to be of a satisfactory size, the fimbriae should be everted by the 'Bruhat manoeuvre'. In this, the serosa 5 mm proximal to the fimbriae is coagulated with thermocoagulation, bipolar electrocoagulation or

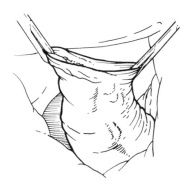

Fig. 6.4 Distal tubal obstruction: the opening is enlarged with forceps.

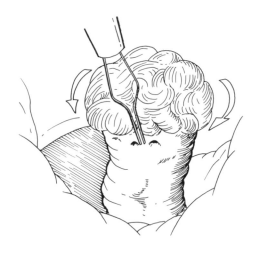

Fig. 6.5 Distal tubal obstruction: the fimbria are everted by coagulating the tubal serosa.

defocused laser. This causes the tissue to blanche and retract, thus everting the fimbrial end of the tube and keeping the neo-ostium open (Fig. 6.5). The treatment of the serosa should be just enough to obtain the 'flowering' appearance of the tube as the fimbriae evert, and not so much that excessive fibrosis and possible stricture formation takes place.

Sutures are not usually necessary in laparoscopic tubal surgery and may be counter-productive in that they may cause small areas of ischaemia and subsequent adhesion formation.

Linear salpingostomy

The radical laparoscopic treatment of tubal pregnancy has been considered a relatively easy operation which can be performed by a surgeon who has been trained to an intermediate standard. Conservative tubal surgery demands more skill and a more careful assessment of the tube and its capacity to function normally in the future. There is little point in conserving tubal function if it is highly likely that a further tubal pregnancy will occur, with possible life-threatening consequences. Nevertheless, the majority of tubal pregnancies may be treated conservatively.

The early diagnosis of tubal pregnancy depends on a high degree of awareness. Any patient with delayed menstruation or an altered menstrual pattern should be seen without delay, the level of serum βhCG estimated and an accurate transvaginal ultrasound scan performed. When tubal pregnancy is suspected laparoscopy should be carried out, and in some 80% of cases this can be done before tubal rupture. Two secondary trocars and cannulae should be introduced through portals placed within the safety triangle. If necessary,

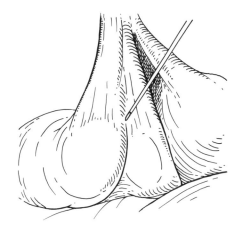

Fig. 6.6 Ectopic pregnancy: Vasopressin is injected into the mesosalpinx.

adhesiolysis and mobilization of the tube should be performed by electro-mechanical or laser surgery and blood clots evacuated to obtain a clear operation field.

The tube should be held with grasping forceps introduced through the ipsilateral secondary portal. It is advisable to inject a prophylactic haemostatic solution, although this may not be necessary if the diagnosis is made early and the tubal pregnancy is small. Vasopressin should be injected in a dilution of 1 : 20 into the mesosalpinx adjacent to the tubal pregnancy (Fig. 6.6). Usually about 10 ml is sufficient to ensure haemostasis. Adrenaline may be used, but has the disadvantage of causing cardiac irregularity and producing vasodilatation a few hours later, with the risk of post-operative bleeding.

If the gestational sac is in the ampulla, the tube should be incised on its anti-mesenteric border at the proximal part of the swelling (Fig. 6.7). The incision is usually made in the tubal wall slightly closer to the uterus than the apex of the swelling because the pedicle formed by the pregnancy is situated at the point. A distal incision

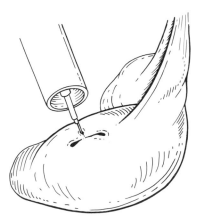

Fig. 6.7 Ectopic pregnancy: a linear incision is made over the proximal part of the swelling.

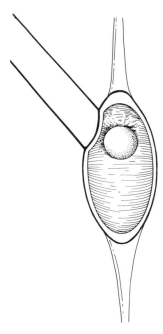

Fig. 6.8 Ectopic pregnancy: the pregnancy is attached to the proximal end of the swelling.

increases the risk of incomplete removal of trophoblastic tissue (Fig. 6.8). The incision may be made with a monopolar microneedle, scissors or laser depending on the surgeon's choice and the instruments available. The opening should be large enough to accommodate a rinsing cannula. The pregnancy may now be dislodged by flushing, and aspirated through the cannula (Fig. 6.9). Repeated flushing and aspiration will usually remove all the trophoblastic tissue but any remaining tissue may be removed with grasping forceps.

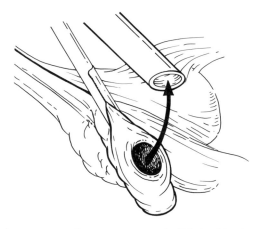

Fig. 6.9 Ectopic pregnancy: the pregnancy sac is dislodged by flushing and aspirated through a cannula.

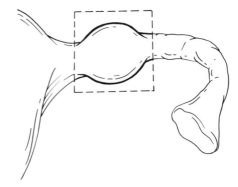

Fig. 6.10 Ectopic pregnancy: an isthmic pregnancy must be removed by segmental resection.

Haemostasis is achieved by bipolar or thermocoagulation of the edges of the incision. When the ectopic pregnancy has been removed from the tube, the wall collapses and the edges come into apposition. Sutures are unnecessary and may tend to increase the formation of adhesions. Finally, copious pelvic lavage is carried out to remove blood, clot and debris.

If the pregnancy is in the tubal isthmus it may not be possible to enucleate it, in which case segmental resection of the affected tube may be performed. The tubal wall on either side of the pregnancy should be coagulated and divided, thus allowing the segment containing the pregnancy to be removed, coagulating the mesosalpinx if necessary (Fig. 6.10). Re-anastomosis may be offered at a later date to restore tubal patency.

Post-operatively, the βhCG levels should be determined and, if the products of conception have been completely removed, the level should fall rapidly within the first 3–4 days. A slow fall suggests retained products which may lead to further bleeding. Ultrasound scanning may help to define the problem, chemotherapeutic drugs such as methotrexate may be used, or repeat laparoscopic surgery may be necessary to perform salpingectomy.

Ovariotomy

The laparoscopic surgical treatment of ovarian cysts has presented one of the major challenges of advanced endoscopic surgery. Physiological cysts may be aspirated but they will disappear spontaneously, so there seems little justification for operating on them unless the diagnosis is in doubt. If there is doubt it is preferable to remove them completely, because pathological cysts will inevitably return unless they are completely removed.

Pathological cysts such as serous and pseudomucinous cystadenomas, dermoids and endometriomas may all be removed laparoscopically. It is unwise to consider removing a malignant ovarian tumour laparoscopically, although a new technique of removing cysts without spillage will be described.

Pre-operative assessment is vital to exclude malignancy and determine the suitability of the cyst for laparoscopic surgery. Malignancy should be excluded by transvaginal ultrasound examination and the estimation of the CA125 level. Tumours over 8 cm in diameter are probably too large for laparoscopic surgery, but of course the experience of the surgeon will determine the choice of route. Laparoscopic surgeons should always be humble and be prepared to proceed to laparotomy if the operation becomes too difficult or there are intra-operative complications. This means that there should always be facilities for immediate laparotomy and to keep the patient in hospital if necessary. The suitability of the patient for laparoscopic surgery must be considered—obesity, cardio-respiratory disease or a large tumour are all possible contra-indications.

The bowel should be prepared pre-operatively to ensure that it is empty to allow loops of small intestine to be retracted out of the pelvis, thus improving access. Antibiotics should be given in case the bowel is damaged during the operation.

Diagnostic laparoscopy should be performed and the ovarian tumour re-assessed before making a final decision to remove it laparoscopically. If necessary, division of adhesions from bowel, uterus or pelvic wall should be performed to gain access to the cyst and to enable its whole surface to be examined in detail. The peri-operative assessment of possible malignancy involves considering:

1 The length of the utero-ovarian ligament, which becomes elongated by malignant tumours as a result of traction on the ligament.
2 The thickness of the cyst capsule.
3 The vascular pattern of the cyst wall, which is more irregular in malignant tumours.
4 The appearance of the contents of the cyst and the internal wall, which should be smooth and without papillae.
5 The appearance of the omentum, liver and visceral and parietal peritoneum, which may contain secondary tumour deposits.

The cyst should be steadied by grasping the ovarian ligament and then aspirated with a suction or Veress' needle. When the cyst wall becomes slack, it may be grasped with forceps close to the site of needle insertion, which will help to prevent spillage of the cyst contents (Fig. 6.11). The contents should be sent for cytological examination, although this is less reliable than histological examination of the cyst wall. The cyst should then be washed out until the contents are clear and a full examination of the interior wall is

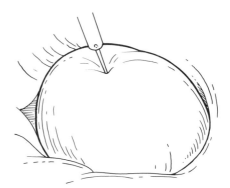

Fig. 6.11 Ovariotomy: the cyst is aspirated with a suction needle.

possible. Lavage of the cyst may be carried out with an aquapurator pump, or simply using a pressure cuff on a saline bag and the operating room suction apparatus. Lavage should be with copious amounts of fluid in the cases of pseudomucinous serous cystadenoma, or endometrioma.

The cyst should now be opened with scissors, microneedle or laser filled with fluid, and the laparoscope inserted. 'Under water laparoscopy' is more accurate than gas laparoscopy when looking for minute papillae in the wall of a cyst and allows the telescope to be brought close to the cyst wall to utilize the magnification of the laparoscope and allow detailed inspection. Small papillae on the cyst wall tend to be flattened by gas and are more obvious with fluid distension.

Access to the cyst to remove it may be improved by using the uterus as an 'internal operating table'. The uterus should be ante verted and the adnexa lifted with grasping forceps. The uterus should then be retroverted and the fundus displaced into the ipsilateral ovarian fossa. The ovary now comes to lie on the anterior surface of the uterus and is more accessible for surgery.

The cyst wall should now be identified and the cyst and ovarian capsule grasped with two pairs of forceps (Fig. 6.12). This is one occasion where it is preferable to have the telescope and camera held by an assistant while the surgeon holds one forceps in each hand and gently exerts traction to peel the cyst out of its bed. In cases of endometriosis, the cyst may be densely adherent to the ovary and must be dissected free with scissors or laser. Hydrodissection may be useful in these cases. This technique allows the cyst to be separated atraumatically from the ovary by water pressure (Fig. 6.13). Laser surgeons will usually treat endometriomas by simply vaporizing the cyst wall and not by removing them from the ovary. Electromechanical surgeons should always ensure complete removal, as

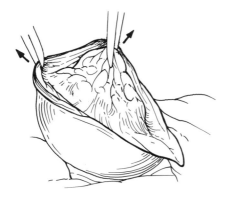

Fig. 6.12 Ovariotomy: the wall of
the cyst is peeled out of the ovary.

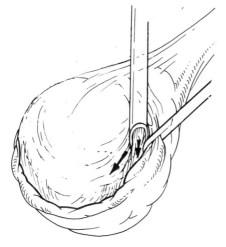

Fig. 6.13 Ovariotomy: hydrodissection helps to separate the
layers.

electrical ablation is not satisfactory. In all cases of cystadenomas,
the cyst wall must be completely removed regardless of the mode of
surgery.

When the cyst has been excised it may be temporarily stored in the
anterior cul-de-sac until it is removed from the abdomen later in the
operation. Before that, the ovary must be closed. This may be
achieved by:

1 Simply coagulating the cut edges of the ovarian capsule and
leaving it to heal spontaneously. This gives surprisingly good results
with minimal adhesion formation.

2 Tissue glue may be instilled into the cyst bed and the edges of the
ovary held with forceps for a few minutes until the glue has dried.

3 The ovarian capsule may be sutured. Sutures may produce small
areas of tissue ischaemia which may lead to adhesion formation, or
the sutures themselves may produce a foreign body reaction and
lead to adhesions. If sutures are used, they should be tied with the

knot buried and the ends of the sutures should be cut as short as possible.

At the completion of the operation, the cyst wall must be removed from the abdomen and submitted for histological examination. The collapsed cyst wall is usually too bulky to go through a 5 mm cannula but may pass through a 10–11 mm tube. Alternatively, it may be cut into smaller pieces with scissors, or a tissue punch may be used to morcellate the cyst and remove it in small pieces. Dermoid cysts or cysts of doubtful nature should be removed in one piece and spillage prevented; this may be achieved by:

1 Enlarging the supra-pubic or umbilical incision and removing the cyst intact. This loses some of the advantages of laparoscopic surgery with its small incisions and the consequent ability of the patient to return home within a few hours of surgery.

2 A cruciate incision in the posterior vaginal fornix allows quite large tumours to be removed without undue upset to the patient.

3 The cyst may be placed in a sterile plastic bag and removed by either route. In this case the cyst may be punctured, aspirated and deflated within the bag without danger of peritoneal contamination.

'Oophorectomy in a bag' is recommended if there is risk of spillage of cyst contents. A specially designed plastic bag with strings at its open end is inserted through a 10 mm cannula and placed within the abdomen. The cyst is then placed in the bag with grasping forceps and the strings pulled through the cannula (Fig. 6.14). The cannula can now be removed, and the incision enlarged if necessary until the neck of the bag comes outside the abdomen. The cyst may then be opened in the bag, its contents aspirated and its bulk reduced. The cyst may then be removed from the abdomen, contained in the bag, without risk of contamination.

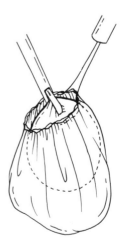

Fig. 6.14 Oophorectomy in a bag: the excised ovary is placed in a polythene bag prior to removal from the abdomen.

Oophorectomy

Oophorectomy may be indicated in cases of breast carcinoma when it may be advisable to remove a normal ovary, as an adjunct to laparoscopically-assisted hysterectomy, in cases of ovarian cysts or tumours where there may be doubt about the simplicity of the tumour, and in those rare cases of streak ovary where there is a risk of malignant development.

Three electro-mechanical techniques are in common use to ensure haemostasis of the pedicle:
1 Coagulation;
2 Ligation of the pedicle;
3 Stapling or clipping.

Coagulation of the pedicle can be performed either by bipolar or thermal coagulation. In bipolar coagulation the ovary is pulled out from the pelvic side wall with forceps introduced through the contra-lateral portal to form a discrete pedicle which is easier to coagulate. The pedicle is grasped with the bipolar forceps and the current passed until it ceases to flow and complete dessication of the pedicle has taken place. This is best achieved using the newest generation of electrocoagulation instruments, which not only indicate the power of the current but also show when the current has stopped flowing and tissue dessication is complete. If coagulation stops before complete dessication, there will be some viable tissue left in the pedicle, increasing the risk of bleeding. The coagulated area is then divided with scissors. The procedure may have to be performed several times until the full breadth of the pedicle has been coagulated and the dessicated pedicle sectioned with scissors after each segment has been treated.

Thermocoagulation is advocated by some workers. Its advantage is that there is less heat produced and no electric current passes through the body, so there is less risk of damage to adjacent organs. However, on the other hand there is more risk of incomplete dessication and therefore of bleeding.

Ligation of the pedicle may be performed with endoloops or by suturing and using intra- or extra-corporeal knotting techniques. The easiest of these is by the use of endoloops. The endoloop is inserted into the abdomen through the ipsilateral portal and laid over the ovary. Forceps are inserted through the opposite portal and are passed through the loop. The forceps grasp the ovary and pull it through the loop, which should then be drawn tight. The forceps

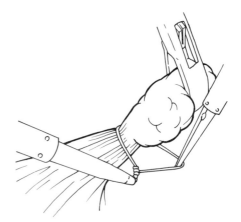

Fig. 6.15 Oophorectomy: a Roeder loop is placed around the infundibulo pelvic ligament.

should be withdrawn and replaced with scissors, with which the short end of the ligature is cut (Fig. 6.15). Two further loops should then be applied, each closer to the pelvic side wall than the previous one to ensure that the pedicle is secure and that there will be sufficient room to cut it without leaving any ovarian tissue in the pedicle. The pedicle is then divided with scissors. It has been suggested that the stump should be coagulated to avoid adhesion formation, although there is no proof that this is effective (Fig. 6.16).

In either technique the ovary must be removed from the abdomen by enlarging one of the abdominal incisions, making a cruciate incision in the floor of the pouch of Douglas and removing it through the vagina or by morcellation. The technique of 'oophorectomy in a bag' as described above may be employed if appropriate.

Stapling the pedicle is now commonly used as part of laparoscopically-assisted hysterectomy when the operation is performed to facilitate

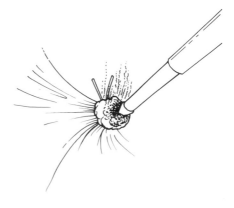

Fig. 6.16 Oophorectomy: the infundibulo pelvic ligament has been ligated and divided and the stump is being coagulated.

oophorectomy. The ovary is again drawn out on its pedicle and the stapling instrument applied to enclose the full breadth of the pedicle. The staples are inserted and the cutting blade pushed forwards to divide the pedicle. This is much quicker and simpler to perform than the other techniques, but occasionally the stapler fails to apply all the staples accurately and bleeding ensues. The bleeding may be controlled by bipolar electrocoagulation. Staples are easy and quick to apply but they are expensive.

Individual *clips* may be applied to the pedicle to produce haemostasis. This should be preceded by dissecting out the vessels because the clips may not hold the full thickness of the peritoneum and the vessels securely. This procedure therefore requires more skill and time than simple stapling.

The Nd : YAG laser may be used to coagulate and divide the pedicle, but care should be taken to ensure that the ureter is not near the line of section as it could be damaged. Use of the CO_2 laser is not so appropriate because it does not coagulate and there may be bleeding, which has to be controlled by bipolar or thermal coagulation.

Myomectomy

The use of laparoscopic surgery for myomectomy is still controversial. The removal of those fibroids which are suitable for relatively simple laparoscopic techniques may not be necessary. Those requiring removal by virtue of their size, symptoms and their possible association with infertility may be too large or too close to the fallopian tubes to be removed safely by laparoscopic means.

Detailed pre-operative assessment is mandatory. A hysterosalpingogram should be performed to determine the status of the intramural segments of the fallopian tubes. Hysteroscopy is necessary to exclude submucous fibroids, which may need to be treated separately or may alter the operative strategy. An ultrasound scan should always be performed to determine the number and size of the fibroids. If they are not numerous, are less than 11 mm in diameter and do not impinge on the fallopian tubes, they may be suitable for laparoscopic removal.

Many of the difficulties encountered may be avoided by pre-treatment of the fibroids with GnRH agonists which have been shown to reduce the size of the fibroid by as much as 30–60%. Pre-treatment also reduces the vascularity, thus allowing safer and easier surgery to be performed with less intra- and post-operative bleeding. Goserelin in a dose of 3.6 mg given by deep sub-cutaneous injection 4 weeks pre-operatively is effective. It may be repeated once if sufficient reduction in size is not achieved. Indeed, the response to goserelin may be such that in cases of fibroids close to the tubal ostium causing intra-mural blockage, the patency of the tube may be restored by the medical treatment, making surgery unnecessary. The fibroids will grow again in a few months but, nevertheless, medical treatment may allow a long enough time for pregnancy to ensue without the need for surgery.

The following techniques of myomectomy are used:

1 Coagulation of the pedicle and excision;
2 Dissection of a deep intra-mural fibroid and removal;
3 Myolysis with laser.

A sub-serous fibroid with a discrete pedicle is the easiest to deal with. The pedicle is *coagulated* in the same manner as an ovarian pedicle and the fibroid removed from the uterus by dividing the pedicle with scissors. It may then be removed from the abdomen in the same way as an ovarian tumour.

Intramural fibroids may be *dissected* out as in laparotomy and myomectomy and then removed. The patient should always have been pre-treated with GnRH agonists for at least one month. Ten millilitres of Pitressin diluted 1 : 20 is injected into the uterus to further reduce its vascularity and the capsule of the fibroid incised with a monopolar hook or knife (Fig. 6.17). The fibroid is then grasped with forceps and peeled from its bed using blunt dissection with forceps or sharp dissection with scissors as appropriate (Fig. 6.18). Bipolar coagulation of vessels may be necessary. It is usually possible to see them before they bleed because of the magnified view obtained by the laparoscope.

The defect in the uterus should be sutured using a curved needle introduced alongside a cannula, or a ski needle introduced through it. The knot should be tied by intra-corporeal techniques or by tying the knot outside the abdomen and using a knot tier to tighten the

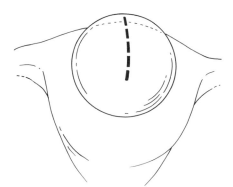

Fig. 6.17 Myomectomy: incision is made in the capsule of the fibroid.

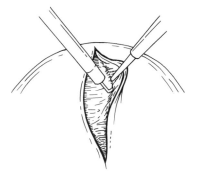

Fig. 6.18 Myomectomy: the fibroid is dissected from its bed by blunt dissection and monopolar coagulation.

knot. The peritoneum should then be closed with a continuous interlocking suture or with interrupted 3/0 Vicryl sutures, placing the knots in the myometrium and not on the surface (Fig. 6.19). Finally, Tissucol may be applied to the uterine wound to prevent adhesion formation.

Removal of the fibroid from the abdomen may present a problem if it is greater than 6–8 cm in diameter. The incisions may be enlarged, a cruciate incision in the floor of the pouch of Douglas may be used or the fibroid may be morcellated with a tissue punch. A more effective way is to enlarge one of the abdominal incisions to about 3 cm and introduce a pair of Kocher's forceps to grasp the fibroid and pull it firmly against the abdominal parietal peritoneum. This produces an airtight seal so the pneumoperitoneum is maintained. The fibroid can then be cut in pieces under direct laparoscopic visual control using a scalpel inserted through the same incision (Fig. 6.20). The pieces of the fibroid are then removed as they become available.

A combined laparoscopic and vaginal approach for removal of posterior wall fibroids has been described. The fibroid should be prepared for myomectomy laparoscopically and the operation completed through the posterior vaginal fornix under direct vision.

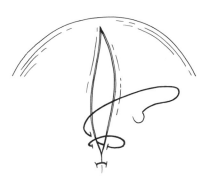

Fig. 6.19 Myomectomy: the incision is sutured with a continous Vicryl suture.

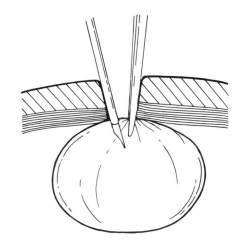

Fig. 6.20 Myomectomy: the abdominal incision is enlarged, the fibroid pulled into it with forceps and morcellated with a scalpel.

Myolysis of the fibroid by laser is now becoming popular. In this procedure the fibroid is pre-treated with GnRH agonists and the fibroid drilled with multiple applications of Nd : YAG laser to devitalize it. The laser fibre should be applied perpendicularly to the surface of the fibroid and introduced into the fibroid to a depth of 5–10 mm. The stroma of the fibroid is then vaporized, removing the laser fibre slowly during application of energy. In this way the fibroid is destroyed without removal. The success of the procedure may be judged by post-operative ultrasound scanning.

Hysterectomy

Laparoscopic hysterectomy was first described in the late 1980s and is achieving popularity as a means of converting an abdominal hysterectomy into a vaginal operation. It must be stressed that laparoscopic hysterectomy does not replace vaginal hysterectomy which, if appropriate and technically feasibile, should be performed without the use of the laparoscope. There may be occasions when preliminary diagnostic laparoscopy is justifiable to make sure there are no pelvic lesions which would make vaginal hysterectomy difficult.

The rationale for laparoscopic hysterectomy is that it is becoming common practice to discharge patients on the first or second postoperative day after vaginal hysterectomy, while patients who have undergone abdominal hysterectomy usually stay in hospital for one or two days longer. There are therefore financial pressures to perform the vaginal operation. The laparoscope enables surgeons to perform vaginal hysterectomy in cases which were hitherto difficult or impossible. In a sense, the pressures of the market place are influencing the choice of operation. However, in addition some of the post-operative discomfort from hysterectomy is a result of traction on tissues, and preparing the uterus for vaginal removal by freeing the upper pedicles laparoscopically prevents some of that traction and so lessens the post-operative pain.

One problem, however, of market forces driving medical choice is that there is a temptation to perform laparoscopic hysterectomy on the 'me too' basis; that is, to do it simply to follow the fashion. The danger of this is that occasionally a surgeon who is not trained in operative laparoscopic techniques may be tempted to perform advanced laparoscopic surgery. If complications occur or difficulty is met, the surgeon does not know how to proceed.

Laparoscopic hysterectomy should be defined as one in which the upper pedicles, broad ligament and uterine arteries are divided laparoscopically, followed by division of the utero-sacral ligaments and opening of the vagina. It is usual to complete the vaginal incision from below and also to suture the vault vaginally. A laparoscopically-assisted vaginal hysterectomy is a simpler operation in which the upper pedicles are divided laparoscopically and the uterine arteries ligated from above or below depending on the easiest approach. The operation is completed vaginally

Indications

The indications for laparoscopic hysterectomy are:
1 Hysterectomy in the absence of prolapse when vaginal hysterectomy is too difficult. This may include cases of fibroids where the uterus is too large for vaginal hysterectomy. The decision will obviously be influenced by the skill of the surgeon in the performance of vaginal hysterectomy.
2 Hysterectomy and adnexectomy where the ovaries are out of reach from the vaginal approach.
3 Hysterectomy where there are adhesions resulting from endometriosis, pelvic inflammatory disease or previous surgery, which would otherwise make vaginal hysterectomy contra-indicated.

Technique

All the accepted laparoscopic surgical techniques may be applied to laparoscopic hysterectomy and to perform it safely, the surgeon should be competent in all of them. Bipolar coagulation or the application of haemostatic clips to the round and ovarian ligaments involves dissection of the vessels to ensure that complete haemostasis is achieved. Sutures may be applied to all the pedicles and tied extra-

or intra-corporeally. These are time consuming and require considerable operative skill but are cost effective. Alternatively, disposable staple applicators may be used which are effective, quick, require less skill but are very expensive. In practice, a combination of the various techniques should be used and the most appropriate should be chosen for each situation.

The first requirement is to be able to manipulate the uterus. This is achieved by inserting a curette or large dilator into the uterus to allow easy displacement in any direction. Special manipulators are available to assist acute anteversion and elevation.

The technique resembles standard abdominal hysterectomy in its early phases and is as follows:

1 Diagnostic laparoscopy should be performed and the suitability of the case assessed. Three secondary trocars and cannulae should be inserted. Two should be placed lateral to the rectus muscle at McBurney's point on the right and a similar position on the left. The third should be in the midline. The level depends on the size of the uterus. Adhesiolysis should be performed to restore the anatomy and mobilize the uterus for hysterectomy.

2 The round ligaments should be divided after clipping or dessicating them with bipolar current.

3 The peritoneum of the ovarian ligament is incised and the vessels defined before coagulating or clipping them. They are then divided with scissors. It is essential to divide the ligaments slowly with small bites of the scissors. In this way, dessication of the tissues may be detected. If the tissues retain a pink colour, the dessication is incomplete and further bipolar current should be applied before completing the division. The peritoneum between the round and ovarian ligaments may then be completely divided to commence the dissection of the broad ligament. This proceeds by division of the anterior and posterior leaves separately, with identification of any small branches of the uterine artery which may be found running laterally in the upper half of the broad ligament.

Alternatively, both the round and ovarian ligaments and the broad ligament may be included in an automatic stapling device, stapled and incised in one movement. It is advisable to dissect the bladder from the anterior uterine wall before applying staples to ensure that the ureter has been displaced laterally. The peritoneum of the anterior cul-de-sac is opened transversely and the vesico-cervical ligaments divided in the midline. The bladder is mobilized by a combination of scissor and blunt dissection. The bladder pillars are coagulated and divided at the point of attachment to the cervix. Difficulties may be experienced unless the correct tissue plane is opened or if there has been previous surgery. It is prudent to instil methylene blue into the bladder pre-operatively to detect damage. In the event of fistula formation, the defect in the bladder may usually be sutured laparoscopically. There is also danger of including the ureter in the tip of the stapling device if it has not been displaced. Stapling is certainly much quicker and easier to perform but the disposable equipment is very expensive, the cost offsetting much of the financial advantages of the operation.

If it is desired to perform simultaneous oophorectomy, the infundi-bulo-pelvic ligaments may be coagulated and divided or stapled as for oophorectomy and the hysterectomy continued as below.

There is some difference of opinion about the management of the uterine artery and ureter. It is safer to mobilize the ureter and ensure that it is retracted laterally to avoid damage, especially when elec-trocoagulation is used on the uterine artery. The bladder peritoneum should be reflected by scissor dissection to give access to the anterior cul-de-sac, followed by blunt dissection to push the bladder down-wards. The ureter can be retracted away from the uterine artery by displacing the uterus towards the contralateral side with the intra-uterine manipulator. The uterine artery should be identified and dessicated with bipolar electrocoagulation before dividing it. Dessi-cation may be performed at a higher level than the normal for dividing the artery during classical abdominal hysterectomy. This avoids possible ureteric damage and adds to the safety. Alternatively, the artery may be sutured with a 1/0 suture and the knot tied with the aid of a knot tier. It may also be clipped or stapled, although care should be taken with the stapler because the staples do not always reach to the tip of the instrument and it is possible to leave a blood vessel outside the stapled tissue, with resultant bleeding.

Depending on the case and the skills of the surgeon, the operation may proceed laparoscopically or be completed by a vaginal ap-proach. Further laparoscopic dissection, coagulation and division of the utero-sacral ligaments may be performed, the bladder mobiliz-ation may be completed and the vagina opened from above. This will result in loss of the pneumoperitoneum but may be advantageous if there is endometriosis deep in the pelvis with consequent difficulty in the vaginal approach. Generally, however, the operation should be completed as in a standard vaginal hysterectomy.

Closure of the vaginal vault may most easily be performed va-ginally but the pelvic peritoneum may be left open or closed laparoscopically by insertion of interrupted sutures or the use of tissue glue to obtain apposition of the peritoneal edges.

The advantages of small incisions and little tissue traction influence the post-operative recovery to such an extent that is possible to discharge the patient on the first or second post-operative day. Her convalescence before resuming normal duties should be similarly short.

Pelvic lymphadenectomy

A few surgeons perform pelvic lymphadenectomy to stage cervical carcinoma and plan treatment. This is a very advanced operation and, in general, should only be performed by an oncologist.

The first requirement is to develop the pararectal and paravesical spaces.

The peritoneum over the pelvic side wall is opened between the round ligament and the infundibulo-pelvic ligament by coagulating and dividing the round ligament and incising the peritoneum with scissors. The medial flap is retracted medially and the pulsating external iliac artery identified. Dissection commences inferiorally and proceeds cephalad to the bifurcation of the common iliac artery. The peritoneum of the medial leaf of the broad ligament is swept off the underlying loose fascia with the closed scissors or the suction cannula until the ureter is reached. There the areolar tissue becomes more condensed and will not peel off readily.

The left and right peritoneal incisions are then joined by opening the utero-vesical fold. The paravesical space may be opened further by identifying the obliterated hypogastric artery where it is crossed by the round ligament 1–2 cm below and medial to the internal inguinal ring. Retracting the artery medially using grasping forceps opens up the space.

Pelvic lymphadenectomy is commenced by removing the fatty tissue containing the nodes which lie lateral to and in front of the common iliac artery. This is easily performed by grasping the fatty tissue and separating it from the psoas muscle and artery by scissor dissection. Care should be taken to coagulate an artery at the cephalad limit of the dissection. This small artery always runs parallel to the common iliac artery underneath the lymph nodes towards the bifurcation of the aorta.

The external iliac artery and vein are next freed by incising their areolar sheaths and gently and carefully peeling the sheath off the vessel. The dissection is usually avascular. The most difficult part is when incising the sheath of the external iliac vein. The vein may be compressed and almost impossible to distinguish from the tissue of the sheath. However, when the sheath is incised the vein may be recognized by its glistening surface. The sheath may be removed from the vein by careful sharp and blunt dissection.

The external iliac nodes lie alongside the artery and are attached laterally to the psoas muscle and medially to the areolar sheath of the artery. The nodes will have been freed from the vessels during dissection of their sheaths. Their attachment to the psoas muscle is released and the specimen may be removed through a cannula or left to be removed with the obturator specimen.

The obturator fossa and internal iliac vessels are now freed. First the external iliac vessels are retracted laterally and the obturator nerve isolated using unopened scissors. The bundle of tissue containing the nodes is then grasped and dissected free using stroking movements of the partially opened scissors. Great care must be taken when freeing the nodes from the internal iliac artery which does not have an areolar sheath like the external iliac vessels and at the bifurcation of the common iliac artery where the iliac veins lie just lateral to the arteries.

Thus it is possible to perform a pelvic lymph node dissection laparoscopically. There are risks of producing uncontrollable haemorrhage, injury to bowel or ureter and there are the problems of prolonged operating time. The procedure has further disadvantages in advanced cervical cancer and ovarian cancer in that it is not possible to perform an adequate para-aortic dissection. However, it is unusual for lymphatic metastes to 'skip' a gland. The finding of negative glands or involvement of only the lower glands therefore may influence the choice between radical surgery and radiotherapy.

Colposuspension

Colposuspension may be performed laparoscopically. The abdomen is explored in the routine manner. A small incision is made in the peritoneum of the anterior abdominal wall and the laparoscope introduced from the peritoneal cavity into the extra-peritoneal tissues. The gas pressure causes the loose connective tissue to separate and an extra-peritoneal space is created.

The laparoscope is advanced through this loose tissue space until the cave of Retzius is entered. Ancillary instruments can now be introduced into space and the bladder and urethra identified. A single suture is inserted into the pre-vaginal fascia on one side of the urethra and then into the periosteum of the superior pubic ramus. The knot is tied by extra-corporeal knotting (there is not room for an intra-corporeal knot). The procedure is repeated on the contralateral side.

A Foley catheter is left in the urethra for 2 days and then residual urine volumes measured until the residual is under 100 ml. The patient may then be discharged from hospital.

Conclusion

The scope of laparoscopic surgery is increasing at such a rate that a list of possible operations is out of date in a few months. In this chapter, an attempt has been made to describe the procedures in which a developing laparoscopic surgeon may be expected to become competent. It cannot be stressed too often that the development of skill must be gradual and made in an orderly fashion. No-one should try to run before they can walk. No-one should progress from simple surgery to the most advanced operations in one step. Progress should always be step by step, preferably under supervision. The alternative is a high incidence of complications and loss of all the advantages of this form of surgery; this should never happen.

7: Laparoscopy for the General Surgeon

CHRISTOPHER M.S. ROYSTON* &
WILLIAM BROUGH†

Introduction

General surgeons showed little interest in laparoscopy until the advent of laparoscopic cholecystectomy. A few surgeons used the laparoscope as a diagnostic tool, but they were in the minority. Since the introduction of laparoscopic cholecystectomy, there has been an incredible upsurge in interest in laparoscopy. The speed with which it has been adapted to provide access to perform the majority of surgical procedures has been amazing.

Table 7.1 shows the surgical procedures which have been performed laparoscopically to date. It is beyond the scope of this chapter to describe all of them in detail. We will therefore concentrate on the more common procedures which are being widely performed.

Cholecystectomy

Laparoscopic cholecystectomy was first performed by Philippe Mouret in Lyon in 1987. The procedure was popularized by Reddick in the United States and Dubois in France and started to become widely used in 1989/90. This new technique has rapidly spread around the developed world. The French and American techniques are slightly different. Fig. 7.1 shows the sites of insertion of the trocars and cannulae and the position of the surgeon and assistants for the Reddick technique. The primary trocar and cannula is always

* Consultant Surgeon, Hull Royal Infirmary, Hull, UK
† Consultant Surgeon, Stepping Hill Hospital, Stockport, UK

Table 7.1 Laparoscopic procedures in general surgery

Oesophago-gastrectomy	Division of adhesions
Oesophageal mobilization	Right hemicolectomy
Heller's procedure	Total colectomy with pouch
Nissen fundoplication	formation
Watson hiatus hernia repair	Anterior resection
Hiatus hernia ligamentum teres	Abdomino-perineal resection
repair	Reversal of Hartmann's procedure
Insertion of Angelchik prosthesis	Inguinal hernia repair
Truncal vagotomy	Femoral hernia repair
Highly selective vagotomy	Varicocele ligation
Post-vagotomy and anterior	Undescended testes excision
seromyotomy (Taylor operation)	Pelvic lymphadenectomy
Cholecystectomy	Nephrectomy
Exploration of common bile duct	Adrenalectomy
Meckel's diverticulectomy	Splenectomy
Appendicectomy	

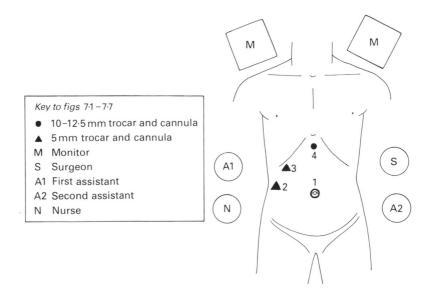

Key to figs 7·1 – 7·7
● 10–12·5 mm trocar and cannula
▲ 5 mm trocar and cannula
M Monitor
S Surgeon
A1 First assistant
A2 Second assistant
N Nurse

Fig. 7.1 Laparoscopic cholecystectomy: Reddick method, the position of the surgical team and the sites of the primary and secondary trocars and cannulae.

inserted through the umbilicus and carries the laparoscope with camera attached. Three secondary trocars and cannulae are inserted. The first allows the introduction of a retractor, which may be a suction/irrigation cannula. The second is used to insert forceps to grasp Hartmann's pouch and manipulate the gall bladder, and the instruments used to dissect and apply clips to the cystic artery and duct are introduced through the third.

In the Dubois technique the patient is placed in the Lloyd Davies

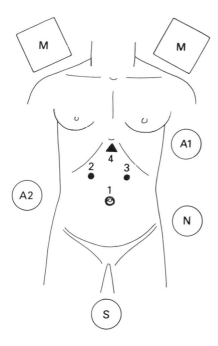

Fig. 7.2 Laparoscopic cholecystectomy: Dubois technique showing position of surgical team and monitors.

position. The surgeon stands between the patient's legs with the first assistant and the scrub nurse on the patient's right. The second assistant, who holds the laparoscope and camera, stands on the left side (Fig. 7.2). In the Reddick technique the patient is placed in the prone position. The surgeon and second assistant stand on the left side, and the first assistant and scrub nurse on the patient's right. In the latter technique two pairs of grasping forceps are used to hold the gall bladder, which allows a more controlled retraction.

Technique of dissection

The dissection starts at Calot's triangle which is exposed by pulling Hartmann's pouch away from the liver. The dissection is performed using either Dubois' monopolar hook, or blunt dissection with forceps. The advantage of the hook is that bleeding is kept to a minimum, but great care must be taken to avoid thermal damage to vital structures such as the common bile duct. If using the hook, the peritoneum over Calot's triangle is picked up and divided using a cutting current. The technique employs a combination of electro-surgery and blunt dissection with the back of the hook. The anterior and posterior leaves of peritoneum are dissected until the cystic artery and duct are exposed. When the dissection is complete, the artery and duct may be clipped separately using titanium clips.

Three clips are applied to each structure: two proximally near the common bile duct, and one distally closer to the gall bladder. The duct and artery are then divided between the proximal and distal clips.

The gall bladder is dissected free from its bed. This can be done either with the monopolar hook, laser or scissors. The gall bladder is removed by dividing the peritoneum on each side of it, the dissection being facilitated by swinging the gall bladder backwards and forwards using the forceps attached to Hartmann's pouch. When the gall bladder has been completely dissected from its bed, it may be placed on the upper surface of the liver pending removal from the abdomen. The operation site should now be carefully inspected to ensure that complete haemostasis has been achieved. If there has been any contamination with blood or bile, copious irrigation is performed and the operation area left dry. The laparoscope is now removed from the primary cannula and inserted into the epigastric cannula. A pair of large grasping forceps is inserted through the primary cannula. These are used to grasp the gall bladder close to the clip on the cystic duct. The gall bladder may now be removed through the umbilicus.

The cystic duct is brought up on to the anterior abdominal wall by traction on the forceps inserted through the primary cannula. The cannula is then removed. A suction cannula is introduced into the gall bladder to aspirate the bile and facilitate its removal. If large gall stones are present, a fistula in ano grooved dissector is passed alongside the gall bladder to act as a guide and the umbilical incision slightly enlarged to allow removal. Once the gall bladder has been removed, final examination of the abdominal incisions should be performed to ensure there is no bleeding. The laparoscope may then be removed. The umbilical wound is closed with a suture to prevent herniation. The secondary incisions are closed either with clips or sub-cuticular sutures. It is important to close the deep layers of the abdominal wall, especially when using a cannula more than 5 mm in diameter. The muscle/fascia layers should be sutured with a dissolving (Vicryl, Ethicon) suture to avoid herniation, which has been reported and may result in the patient subsequently requiring a laparotomy to relieve intestinal obstruction. The patient may usually be discharged from hospital the following day.

Operative cholangiography

Operative cholangiography may be undertaken easily during laparoscopic cholecystectomy. The operating time is only increased by a few minutes. The cholangiogram catheter may be introduced using the Reddick–Olssen cholangiogram clamp, which is passsed into the abdomen through the sub-costal cannula. Alternatively, a specially designed cannula may be threaded through a needle which has been introduced directly through the skin into the abdominal cavity.

There are advocates for both routine use of cholangiography and for its use only in selected cases. The advocates for mandatory operative cholangiography argue that this is an essential investigation to recognize the anatomy and avoid damage to the common bile duct. The alternative group feel that the common bile duct may be just as easily damaged by performing cholangiography if the anatomy has not already been properly defined. The majority of surgeons investigate only those patients whom they suspect may have common bile duct stones pre-operatively. These include those patients who have a history of jaundice, have had abnormal liver function tests, a history of acute pancreatitis or a dilated common bile duct on ultrasound examination. These should be investigated either by endoscopic retrograde cholangiopancreatography (ERCP) with sphincterotomy if necessary, or by infusion intravenous cholangiography. This is to try to ensure that, if stones are present in the common bile duct, they are removed before laparoscopic cholecystectomy is undertaken.

Selection of patients

When laparoscopic cholecystectomy was first introduced, it was advised that the technique be confined to certain groups of patients. Those patients who had had previous upper abdominal surgery or who presented with acute cholecystitis were thought not to be suitable for this operation and were treated with conventional open cholecystectomy. However, many centres with extensive experience now have a policy of undertaking laparoscopic surgery on all patients and the rate of conversion to open surgery is only 1–2%.

Complications

As one would expect, the majority of complications from laparoscopic cholecystectomy occur during the early learning curve. They are most likely to occur in the surgeon's first 50 procedures. The most serious complication is damage to the common bile duct, mistaking it for the cystic duct, or from electric or laser burns. The site of the division or burn, unfortunately, is usually high near the

Table 7.2 Complications of laparoscopic cholecystectomy

Damage to common bile duct
Bleeding
Cystic artery
Liver bed
Biliary peritonitis
Bilomas
Stone spillage
Wound infections

porta hepatis. The incidence of common bile duct damage has certainly increased with the advent of laparoscopic cholecystectomy but, it is to be hoped, it will decrease as more surgeons are safely trained and their competence increases. The complications of laparoscopic cholecystectomy are shown in Table 7.2.

The most common complication is probably a biloma. This is usually a small collection of bile which forms in the gall bladder bed from small biliary radicles in the liver bed. Bilomas cause considerable pain and can usually be treated by insertion of a drain under ultrasound control. Stone spillage is very common but probably of little significance. There have been few reports of stones being spilled into the peritoneal cavity and subsequently causing symptoms. Intra-abdominal infection after laparoscopic cholecystectomy is extremely rare. Infection of the abdominal incisions is relatively common, which is not surprising when an infected organ is removed through the abdominal wall, particularly in an obese patient. If the gall bladder has been infected, the incision site should be washed out with iodine or a similar agent before closure.

Drains

Some surgeons routinely drain all their laparoscopic cholecystectomies. Others use drains for specific reasons. Small drains may be inserted through the 5 mm cannula, but larger ones necessitating a 10 mm cannula are preferable for the gall bladder bed. It is important to use a drain if there is any likelihood of biliary oozing from the gall bladder bed in the post-operative phase. This applies especially to patients who are having laparoscopic cholecystectomy for acute cholecystitis, or if any obvious biliary radicles are encountered during dissection of the gall bladder from its bed. Biliary leakage under these circumstances usually clears within a few days.

Conclusion

Laparoscopic cholecystectomy has rapidly become accepted as the most satisfactory method of removing the gall bladder. It has resulted in a much earlier discharge from hospital, a lower incidence of post-operative complications and a more rapid return to normal activities.

Hernial repair

Laparoscopic hernial repair has been much more slowly accepted by general surgeons than laparoscopic cholecystectomy, and considerable scepticism remains. Techniques have gradually evolved over the last 2 years, from merely attempting to deal with an indirect inguinal hernia, to the present position of stapling a polypropylene mesh over the whole of the inguinal region. Initially, the technique was employed solely for indirect inguinal hernias, merely closing the sac at the deep ring with sutures. In later series, the sac was removed after first placing an endoloop around its base or sealing off the base using disposable staples. A further development was to insert a roll of Prolene into the hernial sac and apply a small mesh at the level of the deep ring. None of these techniques was applicable to direct inguinal hernias and all resulted in a high recurrence rate. The roll of Prolene in the hernial sac also produced considerable groin pain. Inguinal hernia repair has now evolved so that a large sheet of Prolene mesh is stapled over the whole of the inguinal region, thus making it possible to repair both unilateral and bilateral direct and indirect inguinal hernias and femoral hernias. Disposable and non-disposable applicators are now available to staple the mesh to the inguinal structures.

Technique

The patient is placed in the prone position. The bladder should be emptied. Laparoscopy is performed through the standard umbilical approach and the hernial regions carefully examined. A 12.5 mm secondary trocar and cannula is inserted lateral to the umbilicus on the opposite side to the hernia. A 5 mm trocar and cannula is inserted at the same level on the ipsilateral side (Fig. 7.3). If the patient has an indirect inguinal hernia, the hernial sac is grasped and pulled towards the abdominal cavity. Dissection starts on the supero-lateral aspect of the deep ring using monopolar scissors. As soon as the first incision is made into the peritoneum of the inguinal

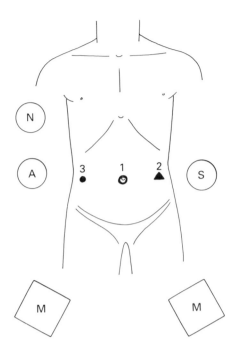

Fig. 7.3 Laparoscopic hernia repair.

region, the pneumoperitoneum gas diffuses into the retroperitoneal tissues and assists the dissection. The dissection is continued to free the peritoneum posteriorly to the level of the testicular vessels and then across the anterior and medial aspects of the deep ring. Care must be taken on the medial aspect to avoid damaging the deep inferior epigastric artery. The hernial sac is then mobilized until the testicular vessels are identified on its posterior surface. The whole of the sac is not removed. The sac is divided and the testicular vessels and vas are freed from the posterior aspect of the sac. Dissection is then continued medially to expose the pubic tubercle and pubic ramus. When this dissection is complete, the testicular vessels and the vas can be seen running up to the deep ring, where they curl medially around the deep inferior epigastric artery to run superficially in the inguinal canal. It is important to mobilize the vas from the peritoneum to allow the mesh to be inserted.

Prolene mesh measuring 12 × 7.5 cm is now introduced through the 12.5 mm cannula and inserted into the inguinal region so that it completely covers Hesselbach's triangle and the deep ring. The mesh is first stapled to the periosteum of the pubic tubercle and the pubic ramus to fix it medially. The superior aspect of the mesh is stapled on each side of the inferior epigastric artery to cover Hesselbach's triangle. It is fixed laterally to the inferior aspect of the transversus abdominis muscle. The inferior aspect of the mesh is laid over the testicular vessels and the external iliac vein and artery, to lie beneath the peritoneum which has been mobilized. The peritoneum is then brought up over the mesh and stapled to the peritoneum above the mesh, thus completely excluding the mesh from the abdominal cavity. Thus a tension-free mesh repair of the inguinal region is performed.

The procedure is precisely the same if the patient has a direct inguinal hernia. Dissection starts at the same place, but with a direct hernia there is no sac to dissect off the testicular vessels and vas and thus the operation is much easier to perform.

At the conclusion of the procedure the cannulae are removed and the incisions closed with a single suture to prevent herniation. The skin wounds are closed with sub-cuticular sutures.

The patients may usually be discharged on the same day. Because the repair is performed on the interior aspect of the inguinal region, raised intra-abdominal pressure will merely tend to press the mesh on to the muscles of the abdominal wall and strengthen the repair, unlike a conventional open repair where raised intra-abdominal pressure will tend to disrupt the repair. Patients can thus return to normal activities as soon as they wish.

Recurrent inguinal hernia

This technique is particularly suitable for patients who have a recurrent inguinal hernia and, indeed, these are often the easiest hernias to repair. The reason for this is that the recurrent hernia can easily be identified by the intra-abdominal approach. The recurrent hernia often has a fibrous ring around it which provides good tissue to which the mesh may be stapled. A further major benefit is that the surgeon is working in virgin tissue, as opposed to the conventional approach where the repair is being performed through scar tissue. The technique of repairing a recurrence is exactly the same as for a direct or indirect hernia. The same landmarks must be identified and the same mesh stapled to cover the whole inguinal region.

Bilateral inguinal hernias

Bilateral inguinal hernias can either be repaired using two separate meshes, each side being dissected as described above, or a single strip of mesh can be inserted to cover both inguinal regions—the 'bikini' repair.

Two 12.5 mm secondary trocars and cannulae are inserted lateral to the deep inferior epigastric arteries. The inguinal regions are dissected on each side. The right pubic tubercle is identified and dissection is continued medially from the pubic tubercle to enter the retropubic space. A piece of mesh 24 cm × 7.5 cm is used. The mesh is rolled into a slim tube and inserted through the left cannula. It is then guided down with grasping forceps introduced through the same cannula to the left groin, where it is inserted into the jaws of a second pair of forceps coming from behind the pubic symphysis. The mesh is then pulled across anterior to the bladder and behind the pubic symphysis until it covers both inguinal regions. It is stapled on both sides to the pubic tubercles and the pubic ramus to cover Hesselbach's triangle, one single piece of mesh thus covering both inguinal regions. The peritoneum is closed on each side and the incisions sutured.

Complications

There are few complications encountered from laparoscopic hernial repair. There is a small incidence of lateral cutaneous nerve injury or irritation. This appears to occur in 1–2% of patients. It may occur from the time of operation or develop after a few days. The patient feels an area of discomfort, hyperaesthesia or anaesthesia in the distribution of the nerve. This is usually self limiting and disappears within a few weeks. Occasionally, a lateral cutaneous nerve block is required to alleviate the symptoms.

A haematoma may develop in the groin. It is usually painless and is felt much more deeply than a haematoma occurring after conventional hernia repair. It may be mistaken for a recurrent hernia. Haematomas may be aspirated by inserting a needle through the skin into the swelling or they may be allowed to resorb with time.

Damage to the testicular artery or vas may occur unless care is taken to recognize and isolate them during dissection.

The main potential complication is recurrence of the hernia. As yet there are no long-term figures to enable us to assess this complication. In theory, the recurrence rate should be low as this is a tension-free repair. The early studies suggest that this will be the case.

Advantages

The main advantage of laparoscopic hernial repair is the reduction in pain that accompanies this procedure, allowing early mobilization and return to normal activities; this is particularly noticeable in patients who have had bilateral hernial repairs performed. Repair of a bilateral hernia by this technique is no more painful than repair of a single hernia and bilateral hernias can be repaired on a day-care basis just as easily as unilateral hernias. It also avoids the complications of penile and scrotal oedema that occur with bilateral open hernial repairs. Recurrent inguinal hernias are particularly suitable for laparoscopic surgery and are likely to have a lower failure rate.

Conclusion

Laparoscopic hernial repairs are still in their infancy. The initial results are very encouraging and suggest that this technique will become the method of choice. Longer-term follow up is awaited to see recurrence rates.

Appendicectomy

Appendicectomy is one of the commonest emergency general surgical operations. For many years it has been suggested that laparoscopy should be carried out prior to laparotomy or appendicectomy, especially in female patients. Often, logistic problems and lack of familiarity with the technique of laparoscopy by the general surgeons has meant that appendicectomy is performed on the basis of the clinical diagnosis. Laparoscopy has the advantage that an accurate diagnosis can be made and the appendix easily removed at the same time. The apppendix should be removed, even if it is macroscopically normal, for two reasons. Firstly, the patient has been admitted with a history suggestive of appendicitis and is likely to present again in the future with similar symptoms. Secondly, it is not uncommon for the histological report of the appendix to confirm the diagnosis of acute appendicitis even if the appendix looks externally normal.

Appendicectomy may be performed in two ways: laparoscopically-assisted appendicectomy and intra-corporeal appendicectomy.

Laparoscopically assisted appendicectomy

Laparoscopy is performed through the standard primary cannula introduced through the umbilicus. Two secondary trocars and cannulae of 5 and 10 mm diameter are inserted as in Fig. 7.4. An atraumatic forceps is introduced through the 10 mm cannula in the right iliac fossa and the appendix grasped and pulled up into the cannula; this places the acutely inflamed appendix and mesentery

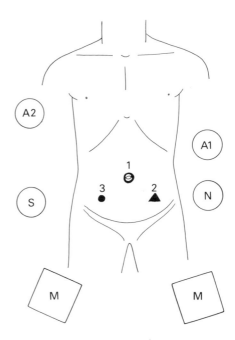

Fig. 7.4 Laparoscopic appendicectomy.

under tension. A fine bipolar dissecting forceps is introduced through the 5 mm cannula in the left iliac fossa and the mesentery separated from the appendix using a combination of electro and blunt dissection. The whole of the mesentery is 'skinned' from the appendix, leaving a triangular piece of fat containing the appendicular artery. There is a difference of opinion as to whether this mesentery should be left after coagulation alone or secured with an endoloop. The latter does ensure haemostasis, although problems with electrocoagulation of the mesentery alone are rare.

After separation of the mesentery, the appendix is usually very mobile and in 90% of cases can be delivered to the surface by pulling out the right iliac fossa cannula with the grasping forceps still attached to the tip of the appendix. When the base of the caecum appears on the surface of the abdominal wall, a traditional appendicectomy can be performed with or without burying the stump. The caecum can then be returned into the abdomen. In most cases, this has to be done by pulling on the caecum with the grasping forceps in the left iliac fossa cannula after re-establishing the penumoperitoneum. The operation site can then be irrigated with Ringer lactate fluid containing a solution of tetracycline (unless the patient is under 14 years of age) and a final check made for haemostasis. The instruments are then removed from the abdomen and the incisions sutured to prevent hernia formation.

Problems

There are few problems with laparoscopically-assisted appendicectomy. Sometimes, the appendix may not be mobile enough to deliver
through the right iliac fossa incision. This may be overcome by
releasing the pneumoperitoneum and switching off the pneumoflator while carrying out surgery on the surface. If this does not give
sufficient mobilization to allow delivery of the caecum then it is very
easy to incise, under direct vision, the congenital reflection of
peritoneum in the right paracolic gutter and fully mobilize the
caecum and right colon.

If the appendix is high and retrocaecal, it is necessary to mobilize
the caecum and then carry out routine laparoscopically-assisted
appendicectomy. In difficult cases it may be necessary to perform
retrograde appendicectomy intra-corporeally. The appendix is separated from the mesentery at the base of the caecum and divided. The
appendix is then mobilized retrogradely and removed through the
10 mm cannula in the right iliac fossa. In these cases the appendicular artery is often thrombosed and does not need to be ligated.

Intra-corporeal laparoscopic appendicectomy

It is possible to carry out the whole appendicectomy intra-
corporeally and deliver the acutely inflamed appendix through the
10 mm cannula in the right iliac fossa. The mesentery is mobilized in
the manner described above and secured with an endoloop if
preferred. The appendix can then be removed using sutures or
staples.

In *intra-corporeal sutured appendicectomy*, the secondary trocars and
cannulae are unchanged. After securing the mesentery, the appendix is enclosed with three further endoloops passed over the appendix in 'lasso' fashion. The appendix is then divided between the
proximal two loops and the distal third loop with scissors introduced
through the 5 mm cannula in the left iliac fossa. The appendix may
then be removed through the 10 mm cannula. The appendix stump
can be buried by a purse string or figure-of-eight 2/0 gauge suture
using a laparoscopic needle holder introduced through the 5 mm
cannula.

In *intra-corporeal stapled appendicectomy*, both the mesentery and
appendix are secured after mobilization using a disposable stapling
device. In this technique, the secondary trocar and cannula in the
left iliac fossa must have a 12.5 mm diameter. A measuring device is
passed through the cannula to determine the size of staple to be

used. This is either a blue or white cartridge which is then inserted into the stapling gun, and passed into the abdomen through the same cannula. The mesenteric vessels are secured first followed by amputation of the appendix and, if necessary, the pole of the caecum. There is no spillage of infected material as both the caecum and appendix are sealed with three rows of overlapping staples. The appendix can then be removed through the 10 mm cannula in the right iliac fossa and the incisions closed. The patient may usually resume normal activities within 7 days.

Conclusion

Laparoscopic appendicectomy allows a more accurate assessment of the patient's pelvic disease whilst permitting the appendix to be removed, without compromising any surgical principles. There is no doubt that the recovery from this minimally invasive procedure is much faster than with traditional appendicectomy.

Surgery of the large bowel

Controversy exists for many reasons as to whether colonic cancer surgery should be carried out entirely laparoscopically. These reasons include insufficient clearance of the tumour and inability to identify all structures, in particular the ureter and duodenum. In addition, at the present time a small laparotomy has to be carried out to remove the excised tissues. However, laparoscopically-assisted right hemicolectomy is being performed with very encouraging results.

Right hemicolectomy

Technique

Laparoscopy is performed through a primary trocar and cannula inserted through the umbilicus and a full assessment of the abdomen made, including inspection of the liver for secondary tumour spread. The secondary trocars and cannulae are inserted as shown in Fig. 7.5. The caecum is then grasped with a laparoscopic Babcock clamp inserted through the 11 mm cannula in the left iliac fossa. Tension is placed on the peritoneum at the base of the caecum by lifting the clamp in the direction of the spleen. This allows the 'double fold' of peritoneum at the base of the caecum and the small bowel mesentery to be seen easily and divided, with monopolar

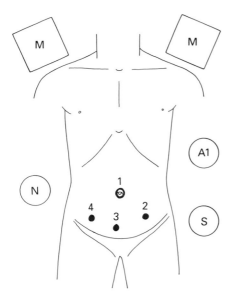

Fig. 7.5 Laparoscopic right hemicolectomy.

scissors which have been introduced through the 5 mm cannula in the right iliac fossa. The congenital reflection of peritoneum in the right paracolic gutter is then easily divided, including the hepato-colic ligament securing the hepatic flexure of the colon. The right ureter is rarely seen and only occasionally is the duodenum ident-ified laparoscopically inside the abdomen. However, it is very easy to enter the correct embryological plane, mobilizing the whole of the right colon in a bloodless field. After the hepatic flexure has been mobilized, and care taken to avoid the gall bladder as it comes into the operative field, the specimen is ready to deliver to the surface for resection.

At this stage, it is advantageous to keep the Babcock clamp on the caecum to identify where the easiest point of exteriorization will be. A small transverse muscle splitting incision is then made in the right hypochondrium. When the peritoneal cavity has been entered, the tumour and colon can be delivered with a combination of the Babcock forceps attached to the bowel and a finger inserted into the incision. At this stage of the operation the pneumoflator should be switched off and the pneumoperitoneum released. When the specimen is on the surface, a normal right hemicolectomy can be performed, but care must be taken to ensure that the duodenum is not still attached to the mesentery. If this is the case, the duodenum is easily replaced into the abdominal cavity by gently pushing downwards until the thin adhesions break down and the duodenum is no longer involved in the dissection. The right branch of the middle colic artery, the ileocolic artery and the smaller mesenteric vessels are ligated and divided. An ileo-colic anastomosis can then be performed in the traditional manner or with stapling devices, followed by closure of the mesentery. The bowel is then replaced into the abdomen and the wound closed. The pneumoperitoneum should then be re-established and the operation area irrigated and checked for haemostasis.

This method of laparoscopically-assisted colectomy allows full mobilization of the right colon without compromising any cancer surgery principles.

Mobilization of the colon can also be carried out as described above and the anastomosis performed intra-corporeally using a stapling device. Although intra-corporeal anastomosis is technically possible, this method inceases the length of the procedure and a small laparotomy is still necessary to deliver the specimen. Techniques will be developed in the future whereby cancer specimens may be removed laparoscopically without compromising cancer surgery principles.

Post-operative recovery

We have, to date, performed 18 laparoscopically-assisted right hemi-colectomies and there is no doubt that the recovery and rehabilitation have been fast. Most patients are able to eat and drink from the first post-operative day and are ready for discharge from hospital in 4–5 days. They are fit to return to normal activities by 2 weeks.

Although the technical challenge of laparoscopic bowel resection and anastomosis has been overcome, these techniques are still under evaluation for long-term results.

Left colon and rectum

Left-sided colonic resection along with mobilization of the rectum has always been regarded as technically more demanding than right-sided colonic surgery and as a result is often left to specialist colorectal surgeons. The same applies to laparoscopic left-sided colonic surgery, in that it is technically demanding and time consuming. Mobilization of the rectum can also be carried out with great accuracy, but is a difficult and lengthy procedure.

Mobilization of left colon

For all the following procedures, the sites of the secondary trocars

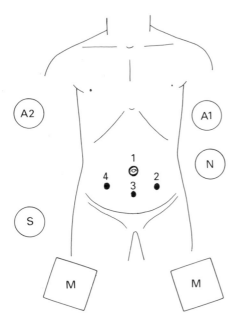

Fig. 7.6 Left-sided colon and rectum.

and cannulae are as shown in Fig. 7.6. The left colon can be mobilized by incising the congenital reflection of peritoneum in the left paracolic gutter. A good view of the splenic flexure is obtained and this can be easily and carefully mobilized so that the dissection enters the lesser sac. As in mobilization of the right colon, the embryological plane can be readily entered and the colon freed. It is rare to be able to identify the left ureter, a problem that concerns the traditional colorectal surgeon. The inferior mesenteric vessels can be ligated and divided, or possibly better, stapled and divided using an automatic stapling device. The remainder of the mesenteric vessels can also be dealt with using a stapler. If the anastomosis is to be performed on the abdominal wall in a laparoscopically-assisted fashion, then most of the mesenteric vessels can be ligated after division of the inferior mesenteric artery.

Mobilization of rectum

The rectum can be mobilized by placing an atraumatic clamp across the upper rectum and pulling backwards towards the spleen, thus placing the peritoneum around the upper rectum under tension. The middle rectal vessels can be seen and clipped. The rectum can then be mobilized under direct vision to the levator muscles and it is then possible to carry out ileo-rectal and ileo-anal anastomosis. The mesenteric vessels can be stapled and divided and thus the colon and rectum can be freed and removed without spillage of their contents. In addition, now that laparoscopic atraumatic bowel clamps are available, it is possible to wash out the rectal stump just as in open colorectal surgery. Depending on the site of the lesion and the indications, the bowel can be brought out on to the surface as a colostomy, or a formal anastomosis fashioned. This technique allows a number of procedures to be performed.

Left hemicolectomy and sigmoid colectomy. After full mobilization of the left colon and sigmoid colon, a small left iliac fossa muscle splitting incision is made and a laparoscopically-assisted resection is performed. The mesenteric vessels can be divided under direct vision or on the surface. The specimen may also be removed at the same time. The anastomosis is performed on the abdominal wall. Some surgeons prefer to carry out the anastomosis intra-corporeally, using a stapling device to divide the mesenteric vessels and the bowel. A small incision still has to be made to remove the specimen and the anastomosis can be performed using an end-to-end stapler.

Anterior resection of rectum. The rectum should be fully mobilized and the inferior mesenteric pedicle divided. The rectum is divided with a stapling device above and below the tumour. The specimen is removed through a small incision and the 'anvil' of the stapler is placed in the proximal bowel. The stapler is then introduced through the rectum and an anatomosis performed.

Hartmann's procedure. The rectum and colon are mobilized and the bowel divided below the lesion using a stapling device. A small incision is made in the left iliac fossa and the specimen is delivered and resected. A left iliac fossa colostomy is then made.

Abdomino-perineal resection of rectum. The rectum is fully mobilized laparoscopically and the perineal dissection is completed in the traditional manner. The bowel is divided above the specimen with a stapling device and the specimen delivered through the perineum. A small left iliac fossa incision is made and the permanent colostomy fashioned.

Total colectomy and restorative proctocolectomy. Both these procedures have been performed laparoscopically. The operation is very time consuming, but techniques are still being developed to carry out this major surgery. For the few patients on whom we have carried out these operations, there has been great benefit as shown by the speed of recovery.

Post-operative recovery

As with other laparoscopic general surgical procedures, there does appear to be a rapid recovery, although this is still under evaluation.

Conclusion

There is no doubt that resection of the large bowel is technically possible and, with practice, will become easier and therefore faster. However, it must be stated that under no circumstances must our enthusiasm for laparoscopic surgery overcome tried and tested surgical principles.

To date, all forms of large bowel resection and anastomosis have been carried out and developments will occur in the very near future that will facilitate this demanding surgery. However, the length of the operation makes most of these procedures difficult to justify at the present time.

Nissen fundoplication

Over the years, many different operations have been designed for the correction of reflux oesophagitis and repair of an hiatus hernia. Several of these techniques can be performed by laparoscopy. The technique which has been most popularly employed by general surgeons is the Nissen fundoplication or a modification of the technique that Nissen originally described. The 'floppy' Nissen fundoplication can be performed very satisfactorily using the laparoscope.

Technique

The patient is placed in the Lloyd Davies position. The surgeon stands between the patient's legs, the first assistant on the left and the second assistant, who holds the laparoscope and camera, on the patient's right. The primary trocar and cannula is usually inserted 2–3 cm above the umbilicus. Four 10 mm secondary trocars and cannulae are then inserted under direct vision as shown in Fig. 7.7. It is preferable to use self-retaining cannulae because dislodgment of the standard cannula leads to loss of pneumoperitoneum. When all the cannulae are in position, a retractor is introduced through

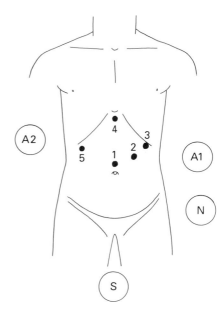

Fig. 7.7 Fundoplication.

cannula no. 5 to lift the liver out of the field of view. When the liver has been retracted, the hiatus can be well seen and the size of the hernial defect assessed.

A Babcock retractor is introduced through cannula no. 3 and the stomach grasped just below the hiatus. The stomach is pulled gently downwards to expose the lower oesophagus.

A gastroscope is inserted into the oesophagus, the light shining through the oesophageal wall allowing its easy identification.

Dissection of the hiatus is performed using atraumatic forceps inserted through cannula no. 4 and monopolar scissors introduced through cannula no. 2. The peritoneum over the oesophagus is grasped with forceps and divided with scissors. The right and left crus of the diaphragm and the oesophagus are identified. Both the right and left crus are completely mobilized and the oesophagus is freed from the two crura. It is particularly important to mobilize completely the left crus and to continue the dissection as far as the gastro-oesophageal junction. The superior aspect of the fundus of the stomach is also mobilized and any adhesions are dissected free at this stage. The right crus is fully mobilized and the tissue between the oesophagus and right crus completely dissected. Care must be taken to avoid damaging an artery which often runs in the superior aspect of the lesser omentum from the stomach to the liver. When the oesophagus has been freed on both right and left sides, the posterior aspect may be mobilized. Dissection should commence from the right side and proceed behind the oesophagus until the left crus is seen. A window is thus produced in front of the left crus, which allows the spleen and stomach to be seen from behind the oesophagus. When this has been achieved, a pair of forceps is placed behind the oesophagus and a soft rubber catheter is inserted to retract it. If the hiatal defect is large, the two crura may be sutured at this stage with one or two interrupted silk sutures. Suturing is effected using a liver retractor inserted through cannula no. 4 and needle holders through cannulae nos. 2 and 5.

The next phase of the procedure is to mobilize the short gastric arteries. The laparoscope is removed and re-introduced through cannula no. 2. The stomach is grasped with a Babcock forceps or atraumatic bowel clamp inserted through cannula no. 1 and its greater curve is held in atraumatic forceps through cannula no. 4. Cannula no. 3 is used to insert scissors and clip applicators to dissect, clip and divide the short gastric arteries. The dissection is commenced fairly high on the lesser curve and continued until 3 or 4 short gastric arteries have been divided and the fundus is completely free.

The fundoplication is performed by introducing an angled grasping forceps through cannula no. 5 which goes behind the oesophagus, the oesophagus being controlled by the rubber catheter round it. The fundus of the stomach is fed into the forceps and brought behind the oesophagus so that a portion of the stomach lies on each side of the oesophagus, which is retracted inferiorally by the rubber catheter. At this stage the gastroscope is introduced down into the stomach so that the fundoplication is not made too tight. The first stitch sutures stomach to stomach on each side of the oesophagus and incorporates the anterior aspect of the oesophageal wall in the stitch. A small fundoplication is made using three or four interrupted silk sutures. When the plication has been completed, the stomach is inflated with gas through the gastroscope to ensure that it has not been perforated. The gastroscope is then removed and the gas evacuated with a nasogastric tube inserted into the stomach. Thorough lavage is performed around the region of the oesophageal hiatus to remove any blood that may be present. The instruments are removed and the incisions closed.

The patient starts a fluid diet on the first post-operative day and may be discharged from hospital on a light diet the following day. Recovery is usually rapid with minimal discomfort.

This procedure is being employed with increasing frequency, but the long-term results have still to be fully assessed.

Summary

These are exciting times that we live in, none more so than in the field of surgery. Over the last few years we have seen a tremendous explosion of interest in the development of laparoscopic surgery and now the majority of general surgical procedures can and are being performed laparoscopically. One can envisage that by the end of the century, the time-honoured laparotomy will be of historical interest only. With the advances in techniques which are being developed, there has come a huge advance in the range of instruments available. Unfortunately, some of the advantages of the surgery are being offset by the cost of these new instruments. If costs are to be contained it will be essential to move away from disposable instruments and return to re-usables, or financial restrictions may limit further developments.

8: Complications

Introduction

No surgery is without risk; complications can occur. The prevalence
of complications associated with laparoscopy is difficult to assess,
because there have been no national surveys since the American
Association of Gynecological Laparoscopists' survey in 1976 and the
British Royal College of Obstetricians and Gynaecologists' survey of
1977. At that time, laparoscopy was confined to diagnostic procedures and sterilization. Only occasional other minor operative procedures were performed. A very few centres had begun to treat
ectopic pregnancies, divide adhesions and attempt salpingostomy.

As operative laparoscopy becomes more widely accepted and
more surgeons adopt this form of management, the complication
rate can be expected to rise. In centres performing laparoscopy,
approximately one third of all procedures are operative but 90% of
the major complications occur in this group. It is becoming increasingly evident that, in order to obtain acceptable results, training
programmes must include supervision at all levels of development
and there must be a high degree of awareness of the potential risks
of laparoscopic surgery.

Complications may be associated with:
1 Failure to complete the procedure;
2 Anaesthetic;
3 Induction of pneumoperitoneum;
4 Insertion of trocars and cannulae;
5 Thermal instruments;
6 Mechanical instruments;
7 Other associated conditions.

Failure to complete the procedure

Failure to complete the procedure is not generally associated with

120

morbidity. However, if the laparoscopy is not completed safely, the patient may have to undergo laparotomy, with its attendant potential for complications. There may be failure due to inability to establish a pneumoperitoneum, or the presence of extensive adhesions. However, the major cause of failure is inexperience of the surgeon or poor surgical technique. The need for proper training and supervision must be repeatedly stressed.

Anaesthetic

Complications directly attributable to the *general* anaesthetic are no different from those which may occur when any type of surgery is performed. As they fall into the purview of the anaesthetist, they will not be discussed further.

The use of a steep Trendelenburg position and the distension of the abdomen may both reduce the excursion of the diaphragm. Carbon dioxide can be absorbed, particularly during prolonged operations. This combination of reduced depth of respiration and hypercarbia puts the patient who is undergoing laparoscopy at increased risk of developing cardiac arrythmia. Monitoring by pulse oximetry, the use of endotracheal intubation and positive pressure assisted ventilation reduce these risks to a minimum. If arrythmia occurs, the anaesthetist will be responsible for its management but is at liberty to instruct the surgeon to return the patient to the supine position, evacuate the pneumoperitoneum and discontinue the surgery.

Vasovagal reflex may produce shock and collapse, especially if the anaesthetic is not deep enough. It may be prevented by efficient anaesthesia and should only be diagnosed when other causes of shock have been excluded.

Local anaesthesia may be used for tubal sterilization. There are possible complications:

1 Anxiety, which may be prevented by administration of diazepam, 20 mg orally about 1 hour pre-operatively.

2 Vasovagal reaction with bradycardia and, in more severe cases, cardiac arrest, convulsion and shock. The treatment is:

    atropine 0.5 mg given intravenously (IV),

    oxygen given by endotracheal tube at a rate of 4–6 l/minute,

    adrenaline 0.5–1.0 ml of 1 : 100 000 solution given slowly IV,

    respiratory and cardiac resuscitation.

3 Pain, which may be prevented to some extent by the administration of non-steroidal anti-inflammatory drugs such as mefenamic acid or naproxen. It is prudent to have an anaesthetist standing by, because about 2% of patients find the operation too painful.

4 Allergic reactions and anaphylaxis. Any local anaesthetic should be given initially as a small test dose to determine if an unsuspected hypersensitivity exists. Obviously if it does, no more medication should be administered. If a reaction does occur it will be characterized by agitation, flushing, palpitations, bronchospasm, pruritus and urticaria. The treatment will depend on the severity of the reaction and may include:

adrenaline 0.5 mg (1 : 100 000 solution IV injection or intramuscular injection),

prednisolone 25 mg IV injection,

theophylline 250 mg (10 ml) given slowly by IV injection,

intravenous fluids,

oxygen.

Pneumoperitoneum

Extra-peritoneal gas insufflation

Failure to introduce the Veress' needle into the peritoneal cavity may produce extra-peritoneal emphysema. This occurs in about 2% of cases. Palpation of the abdomen may reveal the presence of crepitus. If this is recognized early, the carbon dioxide (CO_2) may be allowed to escape and the needle re-introduced through the same or another site.

If the complication is not recognized during introduction of the gas, the typical appearance of extra-peritonal gas may be recognized when an attempt is made to introduce the telescope. It is always essential to view through the telescope during its insertion through its cannula. The typical spider-web appearance caused by pre-peritoneal insufflation will be seen and further stripping of the peritoneum by the tip of the telescope avoided. In this situation, the laparoscope should be withdrawn and attempts made to express the gas. The needle may then be re-introduced through the same or another site.

Mediastinal emphysema

Gas may extend from a correctly induced pneumoperitoneum into the mediastinum and create mediastinal emphysema. Extensive emphysema may cause cardiac embarrassment, which will be diagnosed by the anaesthetist. There will be loss of dullness to percussion over the praecordium. The laparoscopy must be abandoned and as much gas as possible evacuated. The patient must be kept under close observation until the gas has been absorbed.

Pneumothorax

Pneumothorax may result from insertion of the Veress' needle into the pleural cavity. Whenever a high site of insertion is chosen, the needle should be directed away from the diaphragm and, as always, the standard protocol of aspiration and sounding tests employed.

Pneumothorax should be suspected if there is difficulty in ventilating the patient. There may be a contra-lateral mediastinal shift and increased tympanism over the affected area. The procedure should be abandoned and gas allowed to escape. The patient should be kept under observation. Occasionally, assisted ventilation and insertion of a pleural tube may be required.

Pneumo-omentum

The omentum will be penetrated by the Veress' needle in about 2% of cases. The misplacement should be recognized by the aspiration test and the position of the tip altered to free the needle. There will also be a raised insufflation pressure, which should lead the surgeon to suspect an error in the position of the needle. The condition is usually innocuous.

Penetration of a hollow viscus

The Veress' needle may enter the bladder, stomach or bowel. Routine catheterization of the bladder and proper siting of the needle should prevent bladder penetration. If pneumaturia is noted, the needle should be partially withdrawn and the creation of pneumo-peritoneum continued. The bladder peritoneum should be carefully inspected to ensure that no significant damage has been caused. The treatment of a simple puncture is conservative.

Penetration of the stomach may occur when an upper abdominal site of insertion is chosen or the stomach is distended during induction of anaesthesia. Gastric distension may also occur if anaesthesia is maintained with a mask and should be suspected if there is upper abdominal distension or increased tympanism. In this case the stomach should be aspirated with a naso-gastric tube.

The aspiration test described in Chapter 3 should permit early recognition of perforation of the gastro-intestinal tract. It is not foolproof. Bowel penetration should be suspected if there is asymmetric abdominal distension, belching, passing of flatus or a faecal odour. In this case the induction of pneumoperitoneum should be stopped and the needle re-sited to introduce pneumoperitoneum correctly. The gastro-intestinal tract should be examined carefully for perforation. It is important that both sides of the bowel be examined as the exit wound may be larger than the entry wound. Faecal soiling demands immediate laparotomy and repair of the bowel. A simple needle penetration requires no treatment but the patient should be kept under observation.

Blood vessel injury

The Veress' needle may penetrate omental or mesenteric vessels or any of the major abdominal or pelvic arteries or veins. Damage to the major vessels may be prevented by lifting the abdominal wall, angling the needle towards the pelvis once the initial thrust through the fascia has been made, and by inserting only as much of the needle as necessary. Thin patients and children are at particular risk of this injury. It is difficult to prevent damage to a mesenteric or omental vessel, as it is impossible to ensure that the omentum is not in contact with the abdominal wall.

The aspiration test should indicate that the tip of the needle is in a vessel when blood is withdrawn. If this occurs, the needle should be withdrawn, re-positioned and pneumoperitoneum introduced. The laparoscope should be inserted and a careful examination made to determine the site and extent of injury. A minor injury may be treated conservatively and re-examined at the end of the procedure. Bleeding from a major, or formation of a large haematoma formation, necessitates immediate laparotomy with the assistance of a vascular surgeon.

Gas embolism

Intravascular insufflation of gas may lead to gas embolism or even death. This can only happen if the penetration by the Veress' needle goes unrecognized and insufflation commences. It should be prevented by routine use of the aspiration test. The patient should be turned on to the left lateral position and, if immediate recovery does not take place, cardiac puncture performed to release the gas.

Dramatic collapse may result from penetration of a major vessel, but the bleeding may not be immediately evident if it is retroperitoneal. Collapse may also be caused by gas embolism. A thorough search must be made for evidence of the extent of vessel damage. This includes retraction of the bowel to expose the aorta above the pelvic brim, where the most common site of perforation lies. Failure to do so may result in continued bleeding and formation of large haematoma, leading to a second episode of shock some hours later.

Puncture of liver or spleen

The liver or spleen may be punctured by the Veress' needle when a high insertion site is chosen. It may also occur in the presence of hepatomegaly or splenomegaly. The aspiration test and the high insufflation pressure will make it obvious that the needle is sited incorrectly, in which case it should be withdrawn and re-sited.

Complications from the distension medium

Carbon dioxide (CO_2) is the accepted distension medium for all operative laparoscopies. Gas embolism is possible but uncommon because the gas is highly soluble, which allows resorption so quickly that, even if there has been a moderate embolus, the circulatory changes return to normal within a few minutes and the patient recovers.

Cardiac arrhythmia may be due to excessive absorption of CO_2. It is important to monitor the intra-abdominal pressure throughout the operation and to use an automatic pneumoflator. This will cut out if the intra-abdominal pressure rises. Endotracheal intubation and positive pressure respiration will also help to prevent complications from CO_2 insufflation.

Post-operative pain is common with CO_2 insufflation, due to peritoneal irritation which is a result of production of carbonic acid. The chest pain may be confused with coronary heart disease and be treated inappropriately with anti-coagulants. This may produce a wound haematoma or intra-peritoneal bleeding.

Nitrous oxide (N_2O) has become popular with some laparoscopists because it has fewer side effects than CO_2. Anaesthetists can dispense with intubation and allow the patient to breathe through a mask or laryngeal tube. However, in modern laparoscopic practice, a diagnostic laparoscopy may develop into a complicated operative laparoscopy. The surgeon (and anaesthetist) should always be prepared to proceed. In addition, even with good techniques, it is possible to cause intra-peritoneal bleeding with the Veress' needle or trocar and there should always be safe means available to control it.

As this usually means the use of the high frequency bipolar electric current, it is unwise to use N_2O as the distension medium. The only place for N_2O is where laparoscopy is being performed under local anaesthesia and the pain factor becomes important. This is really only applicable to tubal sterilization with clips or rings and not to more advanced laparoscopic techniques.

Insertion of trocars and cannulae

Some of the most serious injuries that occur during laparoscopy are caused by the insertion of the trocars and cannulae. Insertion of the primary trocar and cannula is, of necessity, blind. The site of the secondary portals of entry must be selected carefully and the insertion must always be made under visual control.

It is possible to produce complications during insertion even when the standard protocols have been meticulously observed.

Injury to vessels in the abdominal wall

Superficial bleeding from the incision rarely gives rise to concern and always stops with application of pressure.

Bleeding from puncture of the deep inferior epigastric artery is more serious. The artery is at risk during the insertion of secondary trocars and cannulae. This may be prevented by inserting them through the 'safety triangle', transilluminating the abdominal wall before insertion or by visualizing the artery as it runs lateral to the obliterated umbilical artery.

The diagnosis may be made by the sight of blood dripping into the pelvis from the trocar wound. Occasionally blood may actually be seen spurting across the abdominal cavity. Alternatively, the immediate or delayed appearance of a large abdominal wall haematoma indicates damage to the deep inferior epigastric artery.

The treatment is usually simple. The incision should be enlarged to about 2 cm in length to expose the anterior rectus sheath. A round-bodied needle should be inserted through the full thickness of the abdominal wall from the sheath to the peritoneum under laparoscopic control. The needle point should be brought out again to the surface of the rectus sheath and a knot tied firmly on the sheath. This is preferable to tying the knot on the skin, which is painful and leaves an unsightly scar. It may be necessary to insert two sutures: one above and one below the site of bleeding.

Occasionally, it may be necessary to open the wound wider to locate the bleeding artery. This should be reserved for those cases where there is profuse bleeding or where primary laparoscopic suturing is ineffective.

Injury to an intra-abdominal vessel

Injury to minor blood vessels is usually self limiting or can be controlled by bipolar electrocoagulation. Damage to major vessels is more serious than with a Veress' needle because of the size of the trocar tip and may result in profuse bleeding. Injury to omental vessels may compromise the vitality of a segment of bowel. Treatment of these injuries is by resuscitation, laparotomy, vascular repair or ligation and, where necessary, bowel resection and anastomosis.

A small leak from the inferior vena cava may not be immediately apparent. The intra-abdominal pressure of the pneumoperitoneum and the decreased venous pressure induced by the Trendelenburg position may temporarily control it. However, as soon as the intra-abdominal and venous pressures return to normal, the bleeding may recommence and produce a retroperitoneal haematoma and shock.

It is essential, therefore, at the completion of any laparoscopic procedure, but especially those involving the pelvic side wall, to inspect the course of the major vesels and look for any haematoma formation. This applies particularly to the treatment of endometriosis at this site. Even a small haematoma may be the only evidence of damage to a vein at the sacral promontory or pelvic brim. Occasionally, there may be a defect in the overlying peritoneum which indicates the site of entry of the Veress' needle or trocar. It may be permissible to adopt a conservative attitude if the surgeon is absolutely sure that the injury was caused by the tip of a needle. In this case, the patient may be kept under observation in an intensive care unit. In all other cases it is essential to proceed to laparotomy to close the defect. A vascular surgeon should be consulted.

Injury to a hollow viscus

Injuries to hollow viscera may vary from superficial damage to the serosa to complete penetration into the lumen. If penetration has occurred, the viscus may slip off the trocar, the trocar may remain within the lumen or, rarely, the trocar may pass right through a loop of bowel which becomes impaled upon it. It is always important to inspect the bowel at the axis of insertion of the primary trocar and cannula to ensure that it has not been damaged. If the cannula remains within the bowel, the injury will be obvious by the recognition of mucosal folds. A through and through injury may be missed and become apparent by the sight of faecal soiling, a faecal smell when the pneumoperitoneum is released, or the subsequent development of peritonitis.

Injury to the stomach or bowel is always serious. The management depends on the skill of the surgeon. The classical treatment is to perform laparotomy and suture the bowel in two layers. A skilled surgeon may perform the repair by laparoscopic suturing. The defect should be closed in two layers in such a way as to avoid stricture formation, there should be copious peritoneal irrigation, and a drain should be inserted into the abdomen. Appropriate antibiotic therapy should be instituted.

It may not be possible to identify the site of damage by laparoscopy. In this case, it is essential to perform laparotomy to find and treat the bowel injury. Failure to do so will result in the patient developing faecal peritonitis and becoming dangerously ill.

Minor injuries to other organs are usually self limiting. They should be inspected at the completion of the procedure. Peritoneal lavage must be carried out to remove blood and clot and ensure that the bleeding has stopped. A small puncture on the surface of the uterus may be treated with bipolar electrocoagulation if bleeding does not stop spontaneously. Bladder lacerations may be sutured in two layers using a laparoscopic intra-corporeal suturing technique and a Foley catheter should be inserted into the bladder.

Damage to other organs

Injuries to the liver and spleen are rare unless the organ is pathologically enlarged. Such injuries are more likely to occur in operations performed by general surgeons. Minor bleeding will stop spontaneously. Major haemorrhage requires immediate laparotomy.

Thermal injuries

Burns from electric current were one of the major causes of complications when tubal coagulation was the principle method of female sterilization. The incidence of burns was dramatically reduced by the introduction of bipolar and thermal coagulation and mechanical devices to occlude the tubes. However, the upsurge of operative laparoscopy by a generation of surgeons who have not been exposed to these complications before, has led to an increase in the incidence of electric burns.

Monopolar electric current passes into the patient's body from the electrode, which may be forceps or a needle. The current passes into the patient's tissues at the point of contact and then must return to the generator through the return plate. This is usually placed on the patient's leg. The effect of the electric current will depend on its power and the power density, which depends on the area of application, and the duration of application. To obtain maximum tissue effect, the area of application at the target organ is small. The current passes from that small area along the path of least resistance towards the return plate. In gynaecological surgery this pathway is usually over the surface of loops of bowel. The area of the return plate is large, so the power density at its site of application to the skin is low. However, on its return pathway the current may pass over a small area of contact between two organs. The power density at that point may be high. In this way, a burn may occur outside the surgeon's visual field. Normally this does not happen and the current passes harmlessly to the dispersive plate.

Occasionally, the monitoring system may not be properly earthed. If the current passes through an ECG electrode instead of to the return plate, the patient may suffer a skin burn because the ECG electrode is small and so the power density is high at this site. Alternatively, the current may pass along one of the ancillary instruments which, if not properly insulated, may produce a skin burn at the portal of entry, or the surgeon may suffer a burn on the hands or face.

Bipolar electrocoagulation removes most of the dangers of distant electric burns. The exception is when the monopolar and bipolar generators are activated simultaneously. In this case, the current from the bipolar forceps may pass back through the return plate so that the bipolar system has, in effect, become a monopolar system. It is imperative, therefore, to ensure that the monopolar system is switched off when the bipolar is in use.

There is a danger of lateral heat spread with bipolar current. It is important to ensure that no other organ is in contact with or near an organ to which electricity is being applied.

The bowel is the most commonly injured organ. The injury may range from minor blanching of the serosa to frank perforation. Perforation requires laparotomy, excision of the surrounding devitalized bowel and repair of the defect. If blanching is significant, laparotomy and oversewing of the area must be performed immediately. Failure to do so may result in delayed ischaemic necrosis at the site of the burn. Nothing may happen for up to 48 hours, by which time the patient has gone home. The insidious development of vague abdominal symptoms, discomfort, anorexia and possibly pyrexia may not be recognized by her medical attendants. A faecal fistula may not form for 48–72 hours. Faecal peritonitis slowly develops and the patient may become seriously ill over a period of days before re-admission is requested. Radiology followed by laparotomy reveals the desperate situation. Laparotomy is followed by repair of the bowel or, more often, colostomy and drainage of the peritoneum is required. A prolonged period of serious illness follows and, too often, the patient will resort to her lawyer for final redress.

Equally, or perhaps more dangerous, is the minor burn which may result from direct heat or from current passing back to the return plate or arcing of current from one surface to another. The danger is that these may be out of the surgeon's visual field and may go unrecognized.

It must always be remembered that electric current is potentially dangerous and all the safety rules for its use must be strictly obeyed.

Mechanical instruments

The main injuries caused by scissors or forceps are to blood vessels. Bleeding will be immediately obvious and should be controlled by bipolar or thermocoagulation. Direct inadvertent injury to other organs by mechanical instruments may result from careless or clumsy use.

Other complications associated with laparoscopy

Cervical laceration

It is common for the cervical tenaculum to cause a laceration of the anterior lip of the cervix. The cervix should always be inspected at the end of the procedure. The bleeding may usually be controlled by pressure from a sponge forceps, but occasionally requires suturing.

Uterine perforation

Uterine perforation may be caused by the perhydrotubation cannula or during dilatation and curettage. The perforation should always be inspected with the laparoscope during and at the end of the procedure. Bleeding is usually slight and the complication does not usually require treatment.

Shoulder pain

Carbon dioxide is converted to carbonic acid when it is in solution with body fluids. This is irritant to the peritoneum. Diaphragmatic peritoneal irritation produces pain which is referred to the shoulder by the phrenic nerve. This pain may be confused with cardiac pain by the unwary physician and treated inappropriately.

Pelvic inflammatory disease

There is a small risk of producing or exacerbating a pelvic infection by uterine cannulation and chromopertubation. Post-operative pelvic infection is probably less common after laparoscopic surgery than after laparotomy.

Omental herniation

If the primary cannula is withdrawn with its valve closed, it is possible to draw a piece of omentum into the umbilical wound by the negative pressure so produced. This is usually recognized immediately and the omentum is easily replaced. Herniation may occur some hours after the operation. It is usually easy to replace it under local anaesthesia and resuture the wound.

Explosion

Intraperitoneal explosion is a very rare but dramatic complication. If the bowel is inadvertently punctured, methane gas is released. If nitrous oxide has been used to produce the pneumoperitoneum, the mixture of gases formed is potentially explosive. High frequency electric current may ignite the gas and cause an intra-peritoneal explosion. Nitrous oxide should never be used for procedures in which electrosurgery is used.

Injuries from the operating table

Care must always be taken in positioning the patient on the operating table. Injury can be caused to the nerves of the leg and to the hip and sacro-iliac joints. Compression of the leg veins may predispose to venous thrombosis. The brachial plexus may be injured if the arm is abducted. The hands may be caught in moving parts of the table.

It is important that the patient touches no metallic parts of the table if electric energy is being used.

9: Safety and Training

Introduction

Laparoscopy has been practised by most gynaecologists for the past 20 years for diagnostic purposes and for performing minor operations. The development of more complex surgery has been a feature of the past decade. Few established gynaecologists have had training in this form of surgery and it is still relatively uncommon for residents to have the opportunity of training in their own institutions.

Safety

The preceding chapters in this book have described the indications for, the contra-indications to, and the complications of laparoscopy. A detailed description of diagnostic and operative techniques has also been given. We should now consider the safety protocols.

General

1 Diagnostic and operative laparoscopy should only be performed by fully trained surgeons or trainees under supervision. Skill in conventional surgical procedures does not necessarily confer skill in endoscopic surgery.
2 There must be a valid indication for the operation.
3 There must be no contra-indications.
4 Informed consent must have been obtained.

Equipment

Prior to beginning the operation, the surgeon must confirm that:

1 All telescopes, sheaths and ancillary instruments are in working order.

2 Light sources and cables are functioning and appropriate for the procedure to be performed.

3 Any electrosurgical generator must be compatible with the electrosurgical instruments and return plates.

4 All insulation must be intact and the working parts of the electrosurgical instruments fully functional.

5 Lasers should be calibrated and performing perfectly. The safety precautions for the use of lasers must be observed.

6 The pneumoflator must be functioning correctly and there must be an adequate supply of carbon dioxide.

Procedures

The patient's state of health should not preclude the use of general anaesthesia and she must have no medical disease which would make the production of a pneumoperitoneum unsafe. In cases of pelvic tumours, preliminary ultrasound examination is mandatory to recognize possible malignancy in the tumour.

Local anaesthesia is rarely used for operative laparoscopy. If it is to be used, a small test dose should be administered to ensure that the patient does not suffer from an allergic or idiosyncratic reaction.

The standard protocol must be observed during the introduction of the pneumoperitoneum and the insertion of all the instruments. Preliminary inspection of the abdomen and pelvis must ensure that all the landmarks are visible. If surgery is to be performed on the adnexa or pelvic side wall it is vital that the ureters are identified.

The use of video cameras during all surgery allows assistants to give the surgeon intelligent help. They are vital in the supervision of trainees performing any surgical procedure.

Patients who have undergone laparoscopic surgical procedures must be observed in hospital for a few hours to ensure that there has been no post-operative bleeding.

Attention to these points should prevent complications in standard laparoscopic practice. The first prerequisite to any form of endoscopic surgery is that the surgeon is properly trained in the procedure.

Fundamentals of training

Assessment of departmental needs

The needs of the department will be dependent upon the need to

provide a service, the requirements of the hospital training programme, and the research interests of the department. It may be
preferable to encourage some but not all of the members of the
department to become skilled in advanced laparoscopic surgery,
although it is incumbent on all gynaecologists to be competent in the
surgery of common conditions. These matters should be discussed
and agreed upon by the members of the department before a formal
training programme is established.

Facilities

Provision of the necessary equipment and operating room time for
the performance of complex laparoscopic surgery may put limits on
the number of surgeons who can be trained. Many laparoscopic
operations are time consuming and, in the early part of the learning
curve, operation lists may run over their allotted time. This may limit
the number of surgeons who can be trained in their own institution.
The same limitations may be imposed when learners attend a
training centre. The value of individual training cannot be over-
stressed. An excellent way of organizing this is for the trainer to be
able to visit the trainee's own operating room and teach on a
one-to-one basis. This, however, is time consuming for the trainer.

The learning process

The trainee should be a qualified gynaecologist or a gynaecologist in
an approved training post. The training should ideally involve a
series of steps:
1 *The acquisition of knowledge.* Several excellent textbooks and atlases
on laparoscopic surgery are available. Courses are held in many
centres where the scope of laparoscopic surgery is discussed and live
video presentations are given. These will allow the trainee to
appreciate the scope of laparoscopic surgery. It is vital that the
trainee understands:
    The instruments,
    Principles of electrosurgery,
    Principles of laser surgery,
    Indications and contra-indications and risks of laparoscopy,
    Management of complications,
    The technique of diagnostic laparoscopy,
    Techniques of the various forms of operative laparoscopy.
2 *The skills of diagnostic laparoscopy* are best learnt in the operating

room with a skilled trainer. The trainee should learn the protocol for insertion of all the instruments and the detailed examination of the abdomen and pelvis. Practice under supervision is essential using the video screen to learn the skill of working in that medium. There is no rule of thumb which indicates how many diagnostic laparoscopies should be performed before proceeding to operative laparoscopy. Each incremental step in difficulty should be made under supervision.

3 *The skills of operative laparoscopy* are more difficult to acquire. The would-be surgical laparoscopist must undergo a change in attitude, acquire knowledge and then undertake formal training and practice.

The majority of gynaecologists have been trained primarily in abdominal or vaginal surgery and, possibly later in their careers, have developed an interest in laparoscopy and hysteroscopy. When commencing operative endoscopy, the surgeon must appreciate that the instruments are different from those used in conventional surgery, and it may frequently be difficult for the more senior surgeons to adapt to these new techniques and to accept that they must acquire new skills. Indeed, the more experienced they are at the old operations, the more difficult it may be to change to the new ones, and the learning curve may therefore be longer than for a younger, more adaptable person.

The surgeon must learn to operate in a new environment and accommodate to the two-dimensional image offered by the telescope and then learn to operate from the video screen. The latter technique should be adopted as soon as possible in the training period, as in many cases it is difficult to work without it. In addition to learning to use new instruments, surgeons must appreciate their capabilities, their limitations and their risks. Initially, the staff in the operating room must accept that operations may take longer although, with experience, most laparoscopic surgery takes about the same time as conventional surgery. When the staff appreciate the tremendous advantages of endoscopic surgery to the patient they find it easier to accept the surgeon taking a slightly longer time.

The nursing staff must also learn to use the new instruments and work as a team. This is helped by the use of a video camera so that they can see the operation and assist in its performance. Indeed, their view of the operation is superior to the view they are used to during conventional surgery.

Formal training

The preliminary knowledge acquired at conferences or from reading must now be augmented by further reading and attendance at didactic sessions. Formal training may be acquired by attending a colleague's unit or, if the facilities are available, in the surgeon's own institution.

Before undertaking operative laparoscopy, the surgeon must have extensive experience in diagnostic laparoscopy. At all times, a clear view of the abdominal cavity must be obtained. The surgeon must know when to stop the operation if complications develop, if the condition is too complicated for laparoscopic surgery, or the necessary skill has not been attained. Each step in degree of difficulty should, if possible, be taken under the supervision of an experienced trainer.

Courses

Initially, the gynaecologist may obtain an overview of the possibilities by attending conferences where endoscopic surgery is discussed or, better, where live operations are relayed from the operating room to the auditorium. Video recordings make excellent teaching aids but they can be criticized because editing can make the operation look easier and better than it actually is. Few surgeons will produce a video recording containing the failures of their techniques as well as the successes.

Conferences are organized in many countries in Europe and in North America, either sponsored by institutions or by the instrument manufacturers, to whom much credit must be given for their interest in education and in promoting safety in these techniques. National and international societies are now developing in many countries, which seek to educate by means of endoscopy courses and to monitor the success of the procedures and the incidence of complications. Their meetings also provide a forum for discussion and allow the surgeon who wishes to learn operative laparoscopy to listen and watch the expert at work.

Workshops

Workshops should last 1–2 days and include formal lectures and discussion on the theory and practice of laparoscopy. The groups should be small enough to allow all the participants to contribute and to have the opportunity of hands-on training. Six surgeons is probably the ideal number. In order to benefit from the workshop, they should have had experience in diagnostic laparoscopy and have attended at least one larger conference to appreciate the possibilities of operative laparoscopy. Longer attachment at a training centre may be desirable but not always possible, because of financial constraints and the time involved. There may be inefficient use of time if the trainer has limited access to the operating room, and so a week at a centre may only allow attendance at two or three operating sessions.

Initial training can commence on inert models using a 'pelvi-trainer'. This is a box with perforations in the lid which permit the introduction of laparoscopic instruments. A variety of models may be used. These include pieces of chicken with chocolate under the skin to simulate endometriosis and pieces of liver stuffed in chicken gut to simulate ectopic pregnancy. The exercise of removing the tunica albuginia from a porcine testicle closely mimics the technique of ovariotomy and allows laser and electro-mechanical surgery and hydrodissection to be practised. Inert models also provide the opportunity to practise suturing and intra- and extra-corporeal knotting.

When the surgeon has gained experience in working in a laboratory setting and understands the scope, risks and complications of operative laparoscopy, further benefit can accrue by attending a colleague's operating session and learning on a one-to-one basis.

Having demonstrated general ability, the trainee can be allowed to perform more operations under supervision than are possible in a workshop. The development of surgical skills will probably increase faster and with greater safety than if the learner were to work unsupervised.

In-house training

Some units have been remarkably successful in arranging in-house training. Co-operation is required between the surgeons and the operating room staff. Usually, a week is scheduled so that the didactic part of the course, taught by visiting expert(s), precedes 3 or 4 days of hands-on instruction in the operating rooms.

Practice

The final step in training is practice. As with any newly acquired skill it is sensible to progress from the simple to the complex. The principles of laparoscopic surgery and the details of the performance of simple and complex operations have been discussed in Chapters

4–7. The initial mastering of the skill of operating off a video screen may take a little time. If the learner feels that the time is of such duration that the complex techniques learnt at a training course have become rusty, a refresher course or several sessions spent working with a skilled colleague are recommended before embarking on complex procedures unsupervised.

Conclusion

Diagnostic and operative laparoscopy are valuable safe procedures provided that all the safety precautions are meticulously observed and that training has been logical, thorough and effective.

10: Facilities for Laparoscopic Surgery

Introduction

Day surgery, sometimes referred to as out-patient surgery, is performed on a patient, often under general anaesthesia, who requires the full facility of an operating room and a recovery area but who will be expected to return to her own home on the same day. The concept of day surgery has been accepted in North America for 20 years or more, but the technology and skill to make full use of this type of treatment has only been developed in the past few years. Endoscopic surgery is an ideal way of making full use of the concept: operations which, until recent years, required a large abdominal incision, several days in hospital and a similar number of weeks of convalescence, are performed with only a few hours in hospital and with an equally rapid return to work.

Accommodation

The optimal accommodation is a self-contained unit with its own dedicated operating room, together with admission and waiting area, recovery area and the usual support facilities. The unit is open only during normal working hours and closes completely at night and at the weekend. The operating list should be fully used by a single surgeon for maximum efficiency rather than have a series of surgeons coming at different times during the session.

A less desirable alternative is to use the general operating room and possibly have day cases mixed with in-patient operations. In general, such a unit works less efficiently. The least satisfactory solution is to have day cases admitted to a general ward. The staff are not used to dealing with their special needs. It is more difficult to book their bed in advance and there is more likelihood of their admission being cancelled because of pressures from emergency admissions. In addition, all the financial advantages of day surgery are lost because the wards cannot close at night and at the weekend.

The size of the unit will depend on demand to some extent and the throughput will depend on the type of surgery. For instance, a list of diagnostic hysteroscopies will take less time and each patient will need to stay in the unit for a shorter time than a series of operative laparoscopies. However, working on a mix of cases, approximately 1.5 patients can be operated upon per bed per day, allowing for over 5000 operations per year in a 20 bedded unit. This is sufficient to serve a hospital performing 12 000 operations per year, given that about 50% of these operations may be performed on a day basis.

If the day unit is sited within a general hospital it should preferably be near to the hospital entrance, or have its own entrance, to avoid the patients having a long walk to their transport only a few hours after surgery. It does not need to be in close proximity to an in-patient facility; indeed, many of the best run day units are free standing and the 2–3% of patients who require an overnight stay can easily be transferred by ambulance, even if they have had to undergo an emergency laparotomy in the day unit.

It is not necessary to have beds in a day unit. The patient waiting for surgery can be accommodated on a chair, and then either walk to the operating room or be transported on a trolley, on which she will recover from the immediate effects of the anaesthetic before returning to a chair for her final pre-discharge period.

The anaesthetic area should be of standard size, as should the operating room, remembering that day surgery must always be complemented by the facility to proceed to laparotomy and that endoscopic surgery demands more equipment than conventional surgery. There must be room for insufflation apparatus, pumps, light sources, electric and laser generators, video display and recorders as well as the usual anaesthetic apparatus and surgical trolleys.

In addition there should be self-contained administrative offices, changing rooms for staff and patients, consulting rooms, and adequate storage space for instruments and equipment.

Pre-operative case selection

A decision should be made that the patient is fit for endoscopic surgery and, if appropriate, on a day basis. In general only ASA 1–2 patients (Table 10.1) will be selected for laparoscopic surgery, as the pneumoperitoneum may cause serious embarrassment to a patient with cardio-pulmonary disease. A questionnaire may be given to the patient and her suitability for day surgery assessed from her responses.

Table 10.1 The American Society of Anesthesiologists' classification of physical status

---

Class 1
The patient has no organic, physiological, biochemical or psychiatric disturbance. The pathological process for which surgery is to be performed is localized and does not entail a systemic disturbance

Class 2
Mild to moderate systemic disturbance caused either by the condition or to be treated surgically or by other pathophysiological processes.

Class 3
Severe systemic disturbance or disease from whatever cause, even though it may not be possible to define the degree of disability with finality

Class 4
Severe systemic disorders that are already life threatening, not always correctable by operation

Class 5
The moribund patient who has little chance of survival but is submitted to operation in desperation

---

Operating room staff

Specialized staff who understand the different requirements of laparoscopy and are able to contribute actively to the success of the surgery are required. They must also understand the objectives and possibilities of this type of surgery and be fully aware of the nature of the instruments, their function and their care.

1 The *scrub nurse* supervises the sterilization of the instruments, sets the trolley and checks that all the working parts are functioning, all the instruments which have been wet sterilized have been adequately rinsed, and that the telescopes are dry and have not been damaged since their last use. The scrub nurse actively participates in the operation by assisting the surgeon, having the same view from the video screen. The scrub nurse can increase the surgeon's efficiency by removing and replacing instruments in the operating cannulae, saving a considerable amount of time when frequent changes of forceps, scissors and flushing cannulae are necessary.

2 The *circulating nurse* may be a more junior member of staff who may even be an early trainee and can assist the anaesthetist, help in the positioning of the patient and can also assist the surgeon when necessary, by donning a pair of sterile gloves and manipulating the uterus under the surgeon's direction. A further duty is checking that biopsy material is prepared for transmission to the laboratory and is properly labelled.

3 The *operating room technician,* a vital member of the staff, is responsible for all the unsterile equipment as well as being an assistant to the anaesthetist. The technician also ensures that the anaesthetic equipment is in working order, that the pneumoflators, light sources, video unit, and infusion pumps are functioning.

4 In every operating room where lasers are in use, there should be a specially trained *laser technician* who should be aware of all the regulations regarding the use of laser in theatre and ensure that they are being obeyed. This technician should also liaise with and be trained by the hospital laser control officer and accept responsibility for controlling the laser generator during use and ensuring the safety of the patient and all the other members of staff. The laser technician should have no other duty but to look after the laser during its use.

Organization of the operating room

The operating room for laparoscopic surgery should be as large as for conventional surgery and have room for all the ancillary equipment which is now necessary. There should be multiple electric points situated at strategic points in the room so that there are no trailing wires. The lighting should be capable of being dimmed and there should be blinds on any windows to allow the room to be completely darkened if necessary.

The *operating table* should be capable of being tilted in all directions to allow a variable head-down position for pelvic surgery, a lateral tilt for gaining access to the pelvic side wall, and for the head to be elevated for upper abdominal surgery. The best tables are electrically operated with radio control, to allow repositioning of the patient quickly during an operation without disturbing the surgeon or the sterile drapes. The leg supports must provide various degrees of flexion, from the lithotomy position for hysteroscopy to flat with slight abduction for laparoscopic surgery.

The right-handed *surgeon* will usually stand on the patient's left side slightly cephalad to her umbilicus. On the opposite side of the table from the surgeon there should be a separate *instrument cart* which contains all the electric equipment including the pneumoperitoneum apparatus, light source and video display unit and recorder, and the pumps for peritoneal lavage and hydrodissection. This should be placed near the patient's leg so that it is in line with the surgeon's eye and the operating field. It can also incorporate the infusion sets so that all the non-sterile equipment is in one place and can be supervised by the technician. The *laser generator* may be placed next to this cart, where it is also easily accessible to the technician.

The anaesthetist's trolley should be to the left of the patient's head, thus allowing the anaesthetist room to reach the trolley and the patient without interfering with the surgeon's access to the patient. In many cases the surgeon must lean over the patient's thorax to reach the instruments, and staff should be positioned so that they do not interfere with each other's work.

Lasers

When lasers are in use, there are safety regulations which must be obeyed. Each hospital or group of hospitals should have a laser safety officer who is responsible for inspecting operating rooms where lasers are used, advising staff on the safety regulations and ensuring that they are being obeyed.

There should be warning notices at every entrance and preferably there should be an automatic cut-out which inactivates the laser when a door is opened. All windows should have blinds which are drawn when the laser is in use. There should be a separate gas evacuator to ensure that laser smoke plumes are extracted from the operating room without harm to the staff. There should always be a fire extinguisher in the operating room when laser surgery is being performed.

Care of instruments

The staff must be educated in the special needs for care of laparoscopy instruments. They must be aware of their cost and their fragility and use extreme care in handling, cleaning and sterilizing them.

In *cleaning* all laparoscopic instruments it is essential to remove all organic debris using running water and a soap solution, which lowers the surface tension so that small particles may be removed easily. If the instruments are bloodstained they should be cleaned immediately using a 1% solution of heparin in water which removes clotted blood and tissue proteins which, if not cleaned off the instrument would reduce the efficiency of disinfecting agents. The temperature in the cleaning room should be below 35°C, as above that temperature proteins will coagulate and be more difficult to remove. To prevent scratching, lenses should be cleaned with an alcohol solution and very soft cloth.

All instruments should be disassembled for cleaning and cannulae and sheaths should be rinsed with a water gun to remove all debris from their lumens. It is wise to keep all the parts of the instruments together—it saves time and prevents loss of components. Ultrasound cleaners should be used for flexible instruments and needles. All moving parts such as stopcocks should be oiled daily, and before each operating list the function of trumpet valves, rubber washers, spring loaded needles, light sources and cables and all electrical equipment should be checked. It is too late to recognize equipment failure in the middle of an operation when there is no replacement available.

The sharpness of non-disposable trocars should be checked frequently and the surgeon warned when they have been sharpened so that the force needed to insert them can be reduced. Failure to do this may result in too great a force being used and damage being caused to an intra-abdominal organ.

Disinfection

Disinfection may be produced by glutaraldehyde which has a broad spectrum and acts on Gram-negative and Gram-positive organisms, fungi and viruses. Glutaraldehyde acts by coagulating the protein in cells and impairing their metabolism by disturbing the enzyme processes. It works best at pH 7.5, which is achieved by the addition of sodium bicarbonate. The solution should be replaced every 2 weeks, stored in a non-metallic container and applied for a minimum of 10 minutes.

When instruments are washed with glutaraldehyde, they should be tilted to get rid of all bubbles, all stopcocks should be opened, all protein should have been removed previously, and the instruments should be rinsed thoroughly in sterile water after cleaning. It is vital for the staff to protect their eyes with goggles and to make sure that they have rinsed the eyepieces of telescopes before looking through them.

Sterilization

Sterilization may be performed with:
1 *Ethylene oxide* which acts on DNA/RNA structures in the cells. It is effective at a low temperature and is not absorbed by glass or metal but is absorbed by silicone. It has the advantage that instruments can be packed prior to sterilization, which aids storage of instruments which are only occasionally used.
2 Immersion in *glutaraldehyde* for 6–10 hours, which is an effective

but slow method of sterilization. It is the only practical method of sterilization of liquid light cables.

3 *Steam* sterilization is useful in some cases but tends to shorten the life span of instruments.

4 *Formaldehyde* should not be used.

11: Anaesthesia

Introduction

Diagnostic laparoscopy is a simple procedure of relatively short duration. The anaesthetic can be equally simple. Operative laparoscopy is major surgery and requires the same full anaesthetic technique. The problems specific to laparoscopic surgery, including those caused by the Trendelenburg position and the pneumoperitoneum, have been discussed in earlier chapters. It is not within the compass of this book to consider general anaesthesia in depth, but to discuss briefly the principles as they affect laparoscopy.

Local anaesthesia is indicated in a few procedures such as tubal sterilization and is discussed in this chapter.

General anaesthesia

General anaesthesia should usually entail the use of muscle relaxants, endotracheal intubation and controlled positive pressure respiration. This has some disadvantages for the diagnostic procedure of short duration. These include the potential for minor trauma to lips, teeth or tongue, a longer induction and recovery time and the problems associated with the use of muscle relaxants. In these cases, it is permissible to use a laryngeal mask and avoid intubation.

Operative laparoscopy requires a steep Trendelenburg position and good muscle relaxation. The procedure may take a considerable time, so the problems of carbon dioxide (CO_2) absorption become significant. Endotracheal intubation and muscle relaxants are therefore essential. The choice of drug will depend on the anaesthetist, the requirements of the surgeon and the expected duration of the operation.

Local anaesthesia

Some laparoscopic procedures are suitable for performance under local anaesthesia. These include laparoscopic sterilization and assessment of the tubes for reversal of sterilization. Access to the pelvis is limited by the discomfort of manipulation which increases with time. Extensive examination of the pelvic organs required in the investigation of infertility and cases of pain preclude the use of local anaesthesia for these indications.

The operation should be discussed with the patient prior to admission. She will usually require pre-operative sedation with 20 mg of oral temazepam. Pain relief is assisted by the intra-venous administration of 0.1 mg fentanyl just prior to admission to the operating room.

The standard operating technique must be modified. The patient is placed in the normal position for laparoscopy without head-down tilt initially. The abdomen is prepared with antiseptic solution. At the same time the vulva is gently cleansed. A Weisman–Graves speculum is inserted and a tenaculum applied to the cervix, taking as small a bite of cervix as possible. The speculum is then removed. The Weisman–Graves speculum has only one arm and can be removed completely from the operation field, leaving the tenaculum in situ.

The sites of the primary and secondary portals are infiltrated with 20 ml of 0.5% lignocaine, ensuring that the full depth of the abdominal wall is anaesthetized. While the anaesthetic and Veress' needles and trocars and cannulae are being introduced, the patient is asked to push out her abdominal wall. This provides a firm platform for the surgeon to push against. It also lifts the abdominal wall away from the great vessels. The usual precautions must be taken to ensure that the pneumoperitoneum has been correctly introduced and to prevent sudden deep penetration of instruments. If the secondary portal is sited laterally on the rectus sheath, care must be taken to ensure that the trocar does not skid caudally on the surface of the sheath and penetrate the peritoneum at a distance from the anaesthetized site.

The operating room staff must learn to work quietly and without verbal instruction. The only sound in the room should be the quiet dialogue between the surgeon and patient as each step in the operation is explained.

This form of anaesthesia is acceptable to the majority of patients undergoing sterilization. Some pain occurs in about 3% of patients but it is rarely severe. Pain may be due to the pneumoperitoneum, incomplete anaesthesia of the abdominal wall or compression of the tubes by clips. It rarely interferes with successful completion of the operation.

Index